THE MYSTERY OF SLEEP

THE MYSTERY OF SLEEP

By

JOHN BIGELOW, LL.D.

SECOND EDITION, REWRITTEN AND MUCH ENLARGED

GYAN

Published by

GYAN

Gyan Publishing House
5, Ansari Road
Daryaganj, New Delhi-110002
Phone: 011-47034999, 9811692060
E-mail: books@gyanbooks.com

Distribution Network
gyanbooks.com
India, USA, Canada, UK, Australia, France

ISBN : 978-81-212-6222-4 (PB)
First Published, 1903

2nd Impression 2022

Printed at: Gyan Press, Delhi.

THE MYSTERY OF SLEEP
Author: JOHN BIGELOW

THE MYSTERY OF SLEEP

BY

JOHN BIGELOW, LL.D.

SECOND EDITION, REWRITTEN AND MUCH ENLARGED

1903

"I have remembered thy name, O Lord, in the night,
And have observed thy law."—Psalm cxix.

"The night-time of the body is the daytime of the soul."—IAMBLICHUS

CONTENTS

CHAPTER IX

CHAPTER X

CHAPTER XI

CHAPTER XII

APPENDIX A

APPENDIX B

TO MY READERS

In the year 1896 I gave to the public a monograph in which I endeavored to expose and unsettle, if not dispel, some popular delusions—as I regarded them—about sleep. Of these is the notion that sleep is merely a state of rest, of practical inertia of soul and body, or, at most, a periodical provision for the reparation of physical waste in the sense that a well, exhausted during the day, fills up in the hours of the night. I also tried to give some reasons for my conviction that no part of our lives is consecrated to nobler or more important uses than that usually spent in sleep, or contributes more — if so much — to differentiate us from the beasts that perish. I also assigned what I regarded as substantial reasons for believing that we are developed psychically or spiritually during our sleeping hours as distinctly and exclusively as we are developed physically and intellectually during our waking hours; and that it is, therefore, as much the part of wisdom to so order our lives as to avoid everything apt to interfere with or impair the quality or quantity of our sleep, as in our waking hours it is to respect the laws of life essential to the growth, health, and perfection of our bodies.

Since that monograph appeared I have devoted no inconsiderable portion of my thoughts and time in trying either to further confirm or correct these views, and especially to divine, as far as is possible, the purposes of our Creator in requiring one-third of our lives to be spent in a state of absolute unconsciousness, as in death. The results of such study and meditation have not only strengthened my convictions that the supposed exemption from customary toils and activities was not the final purpose of sleep, but have also made clearer to my mind the conviction that no part of a man's life deserves to be considered more indispensable to its symmetrical and perfect spiritual development than the whiles he is separated from the phenomenal world in sleep.

I have also been profoundly impressed by the abundant evidence that many of the events which occur in the waking hours of our life are governed by the same laws and are instituted to serve, in a degree, the same recondite spiritual purposes as sleep. This has opened what has seemed to me not only a very interesting but vastly important field of speculation. I have thought we might find in lunacy, in idiocy, as indeed in most of the chagrins, discomforts, and infirmities to which all are more or less exposed while in the flesh, an explanation and a use, on the lines of thought, which conduct to what seems to be a satisfactory explanation of the divine economy of sleep; and that all of them, like sleep, are providential interventions to relax the too strong hold which the natural world may have been securing upon our affections.

Adequately to present the results of these studies, and to illume the enlarged horizon which they have revealed, has rendered it necessary to re-write and to so greatly expand the work of 1896 as practically to make a new book of it. I venture to hope that my readers will find in its contents a proportionate increase of interest and importance.

I should be sorry to incur the suspicion of having sought to penetrate mysteries which are meant to be impenetrable, but I believe that the great Creator's works cease to be mysteries when their revelation will not expose them to profanation; nor do I doubt that the mysteries of sleep—like the mysteries of godliness, of charity, of the domestic affections—will be revealed to us just so fast and so far as we prepare ourselves to receive them and carry their lessons into our daily lives. Were they studied with like incentives and by the same class of minds as the mysteries of natural science are now studied, the one would probably seem to us no more mysterious than the other, though the results might prove far more surprising.

It scarcely requires prophetic vision to foresee the time when the art or science of sleeping will be studied as systematically as the physiology of our nutritive and nervous systems, and then much of the literature and pseudo-science now in vogue, relating to both, will find their way into the wallet "wherein Time puts alms for Oblivion."

For the convenience of my readers I will here briefly recapitulate the several propositions which I have tried in the following pages to commend to their serious consideration.

I. It is not consistent with any rational notion of a divine Providence that we should pass one-third of our lives under conditions in which we could experience no spiritual growth or development, as would be the inevitable result of absolute rest.

II. Sleep does not represent or imply rest in the sense of inactivity or idleness, psychical or physical.

III. The suspension of our consciousness during sleep simply interrupts our relations temporarily with the phenomenal world and shelters us from its distractions and fascinations, without which spiritual growth and development—the divine purpose of our creation—would be impossible.

IV. Neither the physical nor psychical changes which we are conscious of having undergone during the hours devoted to sleep can be realized or accounted for if the activity of those faculties, respectively, were suspended.

V. The involuntary subjugation of the senses

periodically to sleep is one of the vital processes of spiritual regeneration, without which such regeneration would be impossible—as is evidenced by the fact that the most important events in the history of our race were initiated during sleep.

VI. The spiritual influence and vital importance of sleep is further demonstrated by the consequences of its privation.

VII. All virtues favor sleep and all vices discourage it.

VIII. The difference between sleep and death may be more a difference in duration than condition. In sleep do we not die daily? Do we not come for a time into the same presences and under the same influences as when we finally quit our earthly body?

IX. Should we not regard every wish thwarted, scheme frustrated, project brought to naught, as a Sabbath of rest, like sleep, to remind us that we are not sufficient unto ourselves, and providentially designed "to withdraw man from his purpose, to hide pride from man, and to keep back his soul from the pit"? Is it not thus that we are taught to regard all our disappointments in life as manifestations of divine love and contributory to spiritual development?

X. Lunatics, idiots, and all persons with more or less unbalanced minds must be presumed to be in their waking hours partially sheltered from the undue influence of the phenomenal world upon them, just as the sane and whole are thus sheltered in their sleep, and protected from evils with which they may be unfitted to cope.

XI. How these views should modify the popular notions of our duty towards the feeble-minded, the unfortunate, and unhappy.

J. B.

THE MYSTERY OF SLEEP

THE MYSTERY OF SLEEP

CHAPTER I

Why do we spend one-third of our lives in sleep?—
Prevalent notions fallacious.

WHY is it that the children of men are required by the inexorable laws of their existence to spend, on an average, eight out of every twenty-four hours, or one-third of their entire lives, in sleep?

Why is their consciousness periodically suspended, and so large a part of every day apparently wasted that might be devoted to the prosecution of the duties which the Author of their being has imposed upon them, or in such innocent indulgences as He has qualified them to enjoy?

Why is this apparent waste made one of the conditions of life, not only to those who are supposed to have been created in God's image, but to the animal and vegetable kingdoms as well?

These are questions which pass through the minds of most thoughtful people at some time in their lives, and, to such as have grasped the great and pregnant truth, that in the divine economy there can be no waste, they are very puzzling.

"Why try to prolong life if so many hours are to be spent in sleep?" asked Kant. He could find no better solution of the question than early rising and a decrease of the hours devoted to sleep—a theory which assumed that all time spent in sleep was wasted.

Most people are content with the theory that we get fatigued with the labors of the day, and need rest for refreshment simply because we are fatigued, as the soil needs fertilizing to maintain its productiveness.

Even science has found no better use for sleep than to repair the waste of tissue; to thus "knit up the ravell'd sleave of care"; and still maintains that one hour out of three, eight hours out of every twenty-four, four months out of every year, and twenty-three years out of every three-score-and-ten are only a fair allowance for that purpose. Such, in substance, would be pretty uniformly the answer that would be made to these questions, and the theory that we rest, and for that purpose only, would as uniformly go unchallenged. Yet such an answer assumes many things as facts which are not facts; and any reasoning upon them, therefore, must be fallacious.

When we say we sleep that we may rest, the question naturally arises, What rests in sleep that does not rest equally in our waking hours? What faculty of the physical or the spiritual nature of man is in repose during sleep? What single function or energy of the body is then absolutely suspended? Certainly not our hearts, which do not enjoy a moment's rest from the hour of our birth to our decease. It is always in the effort to send our blood laden with vital energy through every vein, artery, and tissue of our bodies. The lungs, too, are equally restless in their endeavor to provide themselves with fresh air to purify this blood and qualify it for its appointed use. The process of inspiration and expiration by the aid of an elaborate and complex system of muscular contraction and expansion goes on by night and by day with an unrelenting vigor. The same is true of our stomach, our glands, our kidneys, and of all the other mysterious operations of our digestive apparatus; even our nails and our hair are as tireless as our heart and our lungs. The skin acts more energetically during sleep than at any other time, as the quality of the atmosphere in the room where we have slept, if not specially ventilated meantime, will testify in the morning; and it is in consequence of the more active perspiration going on during these hours that is to be attributed our greater liability to chills during sleep than at other times. Both observation and experiment prove that food taken just before sleeping is digested and assimilated much better than if the man or the animal is forced to walk or run or take active exercise immediately after feeding.

A person in good health, while sleeping, will

expel from his body, by perspiration and without resorting to any artificial means of promoting it, twice as much matter as in the same period of time while awake; and nothing is excreted through the skin that has not been thoroughly digested and deprived of every quality of use to the body it leaves.

The kidneys, too, not infrequently act more energetically during sleep than in a waking condition.

Young plants grow in the night-time, which is also their time for sleep. The same is true of young animals.

Science now recognizes the fact also that every impression made upon the mind of the sleeper produces a change in the volume of the brain. This proves that the various sensory nerves, as well as the spinal cord, are practically incapable of fatigue. The care that man and all animals take when desiring sleep—to shelter themselves from light and noise, to close the doors and drop the curtains, to exclude all disturbing impressions from the external world — teaches us that the whole nervous system—even that of our consciousness, which we are wont to speak of as suspended—reserves its power of action during sleep as completely as at any other time. Certain birds sleep standing on one leg. Water-birds while asleep have a habit of gently paddling with one foot, showing that a group of voluntary muscles are continually active. Soldiers frequently fall asleep on horseback, and even on foot, during a night march; nor is it very uncommon for persons to answer questions intelligibly without awaking or remembering the circumstance. Statistics have been collected showing that out of two hundred college students, forty-one per cent. of males and thirty-seven per cent. of females talk in their sleep. So in our dreams we receive impressions showing that not only the optic, auditory, olfactory, and gustatory nerves are active during sleep, but that the corresponding cerebral nerve - centres are active. Eyes are closed, not because the faculty of opening them or seeing with them is suspended, but simply because we do not will to open and see with them, and this is just what happens with all of us frequently in our waking hours, as when we close our eyes to exclude the light, to favor meditation, or in prayer, and always at night to favor sleep. There is no visual faculty suspended in the one case more than in the other. That our hearing is generally less acute during sleep than at other times is not the result of any suspension of the auditory functions, but, as in our waking hours frequently, from the lack of attention. Any unusual sound, such as would be likely to arrest our attention in our waking hours, is apt to awaken us from sleep. No one can have travelled much on our ocean steamers without remarking the prompt effect upon the sleeping passenger of any unusual noise, though it be far less considerable than the familiar noise of the machinery. Very few will sleep through even a pause in the operation of the machinery. So a disagreeable or untimely odor or smoke will often awaken a sleeper as soon as it would have been noticed by him if awake.

"Nature has no pause," said Goethe, "and visits with a curse all inaction."

People whose brains are most severely exercised are apt to find their most congenial recreations in games of some kind which require a concentrated activity of the mental powers, while no one of them finds it in mental inactivity, not even idiots.

The student when he wearies of one subject seeks his recreation in another. He drops his law or his theology or his astronomy and takes up, mayhap, poetry or music or history. I knew a clever architect who diverted his mind from professional strain by the study of geometry, and always travelled with a copy of Legendre in his satchel. He did not want rest; he wanted change. Milton went to his organ for diversion. Dr. Franklin's favorite recreation was chess, and Jefferson's his violin. Whist and other games of chance, so called, are popular recreations for professional men.

There is a very large number of both sexes, unfortunately, who do little or nothing from one week's end to the other to fatigue mind or body, who yet fall asleep just as punctually and sleep quite as long as the average laboring man. This could not be the case if rest—cessation from voluntary labor—were the only or main purpose of sleep.

It is now pretty generally conceded, I believe, that all the constituents of a human being are either spiritual or material; that what of us is not spiritual is material, and what is not material is spiritual. Fatigue, of course, cannot be predicated of any spiritual quality. No one will pretend that virtue, veracity, patience, humility, brotherly love, are attributes or qualities of which fatigue can be predicated, any more than that twice two are or ever could have been or become more or less than four.

This, of course, is equally true of the opposite spiritual qualities, such as viciousness, lying, inhumanity, pride, selfishness, hate, etc. No man, after feeling benevolent for a few hours, needs to rest his benevolence, and for that purpose become meanly selfish during his repose—a necessary condition either of its absence or its suspension. On the other hand, if anything about us requires repose for reparation or restoration, then it must be the "soul's dark cottage" which the spirit inhabits — our material bodies. But matter has no faculty of initiating or of arresting motion. It is absolutely inert. If matter could be fatigued it could and would waste, shrink in bulk, and perish, if not allowed to rest and recuperate; but no one pretends that the aggregate of matter in the world is capable of being diminished or increased, to whatever process it may be subjected by man. If matter could experience fatigue it might be annihilated—a result which, scientifically speaking, is not supposable; and if any particle of matter could experience fatigue and the need of rest, all the matter in the universe must have the like experience. How upon such an assumption can we explain the tireless energy of the countless planets, which have been dancing to the music of the spheres around their respective suns from the dawn of creation, without relaxing their speed in the slightest degree or stopping a moment for repairs in all the myriads of years? If any particle or fraction of our bodies requires rest, the planets must need it incalculably more.

We shall search in vain for any law, attribute, or property of matter or of spirit which prescribes rest as an end or subjective necessity under any imaginable circumstances.*

* "Throughout nature there is no example of absolute rest, all asserted rest being expressions of relations of bodies to other parts of space. Atomical motion attends all thermal variation; this variation is incessant and universal. Chemical and polar motion is unceasing; and the diurnal and the annual motion of the earth perpetually change the position of every atom of its mass. The interconnected movements of the solar system, and the motion of that system towards a distant constellation, together with the motion of binary stars and of nebulæ, are evidences of continual transition, from which we reasonably infer a motion of the whole stellar world, the verification of which is prevented

When death comes and separates the soul from the body and this corruptible puts on incorruption, matter does not part with a single attribute or quality necessary to its perpetuity and integrity, any more than a house does when a tenant moves out of it; even then it does not rest, but, like the house, becomes as much as ever before the habitation of some other form of life.

Yet every night of our lives sleep descends upon us like an armed man; prostrates us with barbarous indifference on beds of down or straw, and closes up all our communications with the workaday world, as in death.

by the absence of appreciable parallax and by the limited period of our observation. The universe itself is relieved from a sullen sameness and is endowed with activity, whirling life, and beauty, simply by virtue of the never-ending motion of each and every atom."

. . . .

" . . . The balance of the chemist has also overturned the belief so long entertained of the destructibility of matter. Now the conception of its diminution, or expulsion from existence, is as impossible as that of its increase or appearance from nothing; and as the matrix of inherent energy, and representing by its never-ending motion a mechanical force, its augmentation, or annihilation, obliterates all idea of laws of force. It is, therefore, concluded that the quantity of matter and of inherent energy in the universe is always the same."—*One Law in Nature*, by Captain H. M. Lazelle, United States Army.

CHAPTER II

Dreams imply imperfect sleep—Jouffroy—Extraordinary activities of body and mind during perfect sleep—Dr· Hack Tuke on the exercise of thought during sleep—Professor Agassiz' dream—Therapeutics of sleep.

SCIENCE is obliged to admit that in sleep neither the intellectual nor moral faculties are at rest all the time. The voluminous history of dreams, somnambulism, hypnotism, quasi - supernatural exhibitions of memory, of courage, and of moral susceptibility, must all be accounted for before the dogma of sleep can be accepted as implying at any moment a state of absolute rest for our spiritual any more than for our material natures —for our souls than for our bodies.

"I have never been able to comprehend," says Jouffroy, "what people mean who say that the mind sleeps. It is impossible to show that in sleep there are moments when the mind does not dream. Having no recollection of these dreams does not prove that we have not dreamed.

"It will not be questioned that the mind is sometimes awake while the senses sleep.

"The fact that the mind sometimes sleeps with the senses is not established. All the analogies go to prove that the mind is always awake. Conflicting facts are required to destroy this inference; but all facts, on the contrary, seem to confirm it. To me they imply this conclusion—that the mind during sleep is not in a special mood or state, *but that it goes on and develops itself absolutely as in the waking hours.*"*

A rustic visiting a large city for a night or two finds it difficult to sleep. A person reading a book finds it difficult to fix his attention while conversation is going on around him. After a while the novelty of these distractions wears off and fails to demand or receive any attention. Evidently the distraction in either case was not an affair of the senses, but purely of the mind.

It is not the senses that first hear the noises of the street or of the salon annoyingly, and gradually less, and finally not at all; it is the attention of the mind which is occupied with or neglects these sensations. The same sounds only render the savage and the blind man more sensible of them; but, on the other hand, familiarity with the sounds renders the rustic in town constantly more insensible to them.

Were the effect physical, and dependent on the body and not on the mind, this action would be contrary and logically impossible; for either the habit weakens the physical organ or sharpens

* Jouffroy, *Mélanges Philosophiques du Sommeil.*

it. It could not yield both these results at once, as it does in the case we have supposed of the savage and the blind.

The fact is that it neither weakens nor sharpens the sensibility of the organ, which receives always the same sensations; but when these sensations interest or concern us the mind takes a note of and analyzes them. When they cease to interest or concern us the mind gets accustomed gradually to neglect them and does not analyze them.

The phenomenon is purely psychical, not physical. The noise being the same on the hundredth day of the rustic's sojourn in the city as the first, the difference in the effect can only be in the mind. Had the soul slept with the body it would have been equally put to sleep in both cases, and one would see no reason for either awakening rather than the other.

These facts seem to amount to a demonstration that the mind does not sleep like the body, but, disquieted by unaccustomed sensations, it awakens, and when those sensations become familiar, they do not awaken it.

There is an explanation of this difference which only confirms its correctness. If the mind be disquieted by unusual noises it has need of the senses to inform it of the cause and to relieve it from its inquietude. It is that which obliges it to awake; hence we find ourselves disquieted by an extraordinary noise, which would not have happened had not our minds been aroused by this noise before we awoke.

There is but one explanation of this. The soul or mind which watches knows whence come the sensations, and does not disquiet itself nor awaken the sensations to report on them unless they are unfamiliar and involve some duty to be performed or evil to be avoided. The unusual noise of a maid sweeping the carpet in a room adjoining your chamber, though comparatively feeble, will awaken the sleeper, while the whistle of a railway train which may be heard for miles, but to which he is inured, will not disturb him. So a nurse will sleep through all noises which do not concern her patient, while he cannot turn in his bed, nor draw a sigh, or even exhibit an unusual respiration, without attracting her attention.

So also we may be quite sure of awakening at a fixed hour if on the previous evening we resolve to do so; but if we rely upon others to awaken us we lose the faculty. The mind is our alarm-clock, which, if properly set, rarely deceives us. The senses are merely the instruments which obey the directions of the mind.

The experience of the Scotch ploughboy who complained that he never enjoyed a night's rest because as soon as he put his head on his pillow it was time to get up again, is an experience by no means rare, especially among the young who live a good deal in the open air and indulge no habits to interfere with sleep.

The reader's attention will now be invited to some other phenomena which are inconsistent with the idea that sleep is a condition of absolute repose, and which science neither attempts to gainsay nor explain.

Dreams ordinarily imply more or less imperfect sleep; a partial interruption only of our relations with external objects; the twilight or dawn of the phenomenal world as we are just entering it in the morning or just leaving it at night.

As Robert Herrick sings:

> "Here we are all by day; by night we're hurled
> By dreams each one into a several world."

They are to the sleeper what the shore is to the swimmer when, emerging from the sea, his feet get support from the earthly bottom. Of the dreams—or, rather, of the mental or spiritual operations which we experience between this twilight and dawn;—that is, while our sleep is profound—our memory takes no note. We are only conscious of dreams which occur when the phenomenal world is only partially excluded from our consciousness; when we are, as it were, mounting the shore from the deep waters in which our souls have been immersed. Hence, perhaps, the confused, inconsequential, and fantastic character of what we can recall of most of them. The presumption, therefore, is that what takes place in our profound sleep, which is not in the least degree adulterated by direct influences from the phenomenal world, is entirely free from what seems often so improbable and fantastic in our remembered dreams—which are obviously a medley of emanations from two widely different worlds or states of being.*

All dreaming, as distinguished from sleep, is imperfect sleep; it is a condition in which the phenomenal world has already begun to dawn upon us again. Our consciousness, of course, returns with it, *pari passu*. One never remembers a dream without waking, nor is one conscious of dreaming until partially awake. Jouffroy was very right in affirming that our minds were active in sleep as at other times; but neither facts nor logic will support the contention "that we never sleep without dreaming."

The sleep-walker, or somnambulist, exhibits at times even more vitality and energy than he would be capable of exhibiting in a waking state. He not only walks, runs, rides, and does other things which he is accustomed to do, but with his eyes entirely closed he seems to have perceptions supernaturally acute. He walks with confidence and safety along the roofs of houses, on the banks of rivers, and other perilous places, where nothing could have tempted him to go

* In the citation above given from his writings Jouffroy confounds the impressions made in dreams, of which we are more or less conscious, with impressions received in profound sleep, of which we are rarely, if ever, conscious except through divine permission.

when awake. What is more marvellous, he will write with critical accuracy in prose and verse; he will compose music; he will choose from among many specimens those best adapted to the most delicate work, with a promptness and precision of which, when awake, he would be wholly incapable.

"That the exercise of thought—and this on a high level—is consistent with sleep can hardly be doubted," says Dr. Hack Tuke, an eminent English authority. "Arguments are employed in debate which are not always illogical. We dreamed one night, subsequent to a lively conversation with a friend on spiritualism, that we instituted a number of test experiments in reference to it. The nature of these tests was retained vividly in the memory after waking. They were by no means wanting in ingenuity, and proved that the mental operations were in good form.

"That the higher moral sentiments are called into action in some instances must be admitted by those who take the trouble to analyze the motives by which they have been actuated during sleep. The conscience may be as loud in its calls and reproofs in the night as in the day.

"The memory, freed from distraction as it sometimes is, is so vivid as to enable the sleeper to recall events which had happened years before and which had been entirely forgotten.

"The dreamer is free from the nervousness

or lack of courage or dread of the opinion of others from which he may suffer during the waking state."*

It deserves to be noted here that neither mesmerism, animal magnetism, hypnotism, nor any of the modern forms of super-normal or voluntary sleep can with propriety be attributed to what are commonly regarded as the chief and normal provocatives of sleep—fatigue and exhaustion.

It is also to be noted that all are used to a greater or less extent in the treatment of disease and as a part of the curriculum of the most important medical schools in the world.

In artificial sleep there may be exhibited the same evidences of languor and fatigue. Hypnosis may be induced by presenting to the hypnotic any one idea or image either by speech or example, as by stimulating the organs of vision or of hearing or of touch, by the ticking of a watch, a monotonous song or lullaby, or by gently stroking the skin. In every one of these cases the attention of the hypnotic is concentrated to a single object, and gradually detached from all else of the phenomenal world. This is the one uniform characteristic, I believe, of all hypnotic, mesmeric, and lethargic conditions whenever, wherever, and however induced.

The reader will please to bear in mind that absolute detachment from the phenomenal world

* Dr. Hack Tuke, *Medical Physiology of Dreams.*

is the uniform condition of sleep, however provoked or incited. I hope later to further illustrate the enormous importance of this principle.

If, as it is no presumption to assume, there is nothing of divine ordinance that goes to waste, there must be a purpose in this periodical and universal change which we call sleep, conceived in infinite wisdom, and of course, therefore, for an infinitely important purpose, and what we call rest is only an incident, and certainly cannot be that ultimate purpose.

What, then, is that ultimate purpose?

If we will reason from what we know, or easily can know; if we will resist the propensity to confound material phenomena with mental and spiritual operations, and keep distinctly before our minds, to the best of our comprehension, the ends or final purpose of our birth and experiences in this world, need we despair of obtaining a satisfactory solution of all these problems, without ascribing to matter or to spirit attributes which neither possesses, and without any wayward or presumptuous interpretation of the ways of God to men?

May we not be permitted to extort some further information about the uses and results of so many activities as are going on within us while in a state of presumed entire inactivity; some explanation of the daily and extraordinary improvement in our mental, our moral, and our physical condition, which no amount or kind of labor by day, when all our faculties are assumed to be at their best, ever yields?

The late Professor Agassiz, in one of his scientific works, relates a very curious dream, interesting not only as a psychological fact, but as illustrating the indefatigable activity of the human mind. I give it as it has been reported by his widow in her biography of her distinguished husband.*

"He had been for two weeks striving to decipher the somewhat obscure impression of a fossil fish on the stone slab in which it was preserved. Weary and perplexed, he put his work aside at last, and tried to dismiss it from his mind. Shortly after, he waked one night persuaded that while asleep he had seen his fish with all the missing features perfectly restored. But when he tried to hold and make fast the image it escaped him. Nevertheless, he went early to the Jardin des Plantes, thinking that on looking anew at the impression he should see something which would put him on the track of his vision. In vain—the blurred record was as blank as ever. The next night he saw the fish again, but with no more satisfactory result. When he awoke it disappeared from his memory as before. Hoping that the same experience might be repeated, on the third night he placed a pencil and paper beside his bed before going to sleep.

"Accordingly, towards morning the fish reappeared in his dream, confusedly at first, but at last with such distinctness that he had no longer any doubt as to its

* *Recherches sur les Poissons Fossiles.* "Cyclopoma Spinosum Agassiz." Vol. iv. tab. i. pp. 20, 21.

zoological characters. Still half dreaming, in perfect darkness, he traced these characters on the sheet of paper at the bedside. In the morning he was surprised to see in his nocturnal sketch features which he thought it impossible the fossil itself should reveal. He hastened to the Jardin des Plantes, and, with his drawing as a guide, succeeded in chiselling away the surface of the stone under which portions of the fish proved to be hidden. When wholly exposed it corresponded with his dream and his drawing, and he succeeded in classifying it with ease."

CHAPTER III

Sleep interrupts all conscious relations with the phenomenal world, and thus becomes one of the vital processes of spiritual regeneration — Nocturnal darkness an ally of sleep—Our transformation in sleep—Lucretius—Bryant's "Land of Dreams"—Voltaire—Venerable Bede—Swedenborg as a seer.

THE first and most impressive fact of universal experience that we note as an incident of sleep is our sudden and complete dissociation from the world in which we live; the interruption of all conscious relations with matters which engross our attention during our waking hours. No matter how much we are absorbed by private or public affairs, no matter how vast the worldly interests that seem to be depending upon every waking hour, with what cares we are perplexed, what aspirations we indulge, they can postpone but a few hours at most the visit of this inexorable master, while they cannot diminish in the slightest degree the lawful measure of his exactions. Sleep, like death, knocks at the doors of kings' palaces as well as poor men's cottages. It is no respecter of persons, and while it is levying its tribute we are unconscious of everything we have done in the past and of all we were planning to do in the future.

Here we have one of the universal conditions of sleep which is coincident and in harmony with one of the supreme behests of a Christian life: utter deliverance from the domination of the phenomenal world; an entire emancipation, for these few sleeping hours, from the cares and ambitions of the life into which we were born, and to the indulgence of which we are inclined by nature to surrender the service of all our vital energies. If it be a good thing to live above the world, to regard our phenomenal life as transitory, as designed merely or mainly to educate us for a more elevated existence, to serve us as a means, not an end, then we have in sleep, apparently, an ally and coadjutor—at least to the extent of periodically delivering us from a servile dependence upon what ought to be a good slave, but is always a bad master. We here recognize an incontestable analogy at least between the phenomena of sleep and the providential process by which the regeneration of the human soul is to be begun, and by which only such regeneration can be successfully prosecuted. The very existence of such an analogy is a fact of immeasurable interest and importance, for such analogies in the scheme of divine government are not accidental; are not without a purpose proportioned to the dignity of their august origin.

There are certain provisions of nature which

may be justly regarded as auxiliaries to sleep and universal in their operation. At uniform intervals in every twenty-four hours of our life the sun withdraws its light and covers most of the habitable portions of our planet with a mantle of darkness. This not only invites sleep by withholding a stimulus which discourages it, but practically interrupts or modifies all forms of industrial activity; it interferes seriously with locomotion; it suspends most of the plans and occupations which engage our attention during the sunlit hours of the day, and emancipates us for a few hours of every day from the dominion of our natural propensities and passions, which engross so much of our time and thought by day.

Nor is it only by the setting of the sun that we are invited daily to give pause for a few hours to our worldly strifes.

In sleep all the sensorial and other functions dependent upon or under the government of the will are relaxed. To secure this relaxation, we seek positions, places, and all other conditions best calculated to shelter us from light, noise, and all other awakening influences. Like man, the lower animals at such times choose a retired place, assume postures which demand no voluntary effort and which expose them least to the external forces which may chance to environ them. The serpent coils himself up so as to expose as little superficial surface as possible to disturbance; the bird conceals his head under his wing; the porcupine covers his eyes with his tail; the skunk rolls himself into a ball; the dog covers his face with his paw.

Why should the ploughman leave his plough in its furrow when the sun ceases to light his way? Can any other more satisfactory reason be suggested than that he may for a few hours be as one dead to the concerns of his farm and plough, and his soul for a time be freed from their distractions? Whatever else may be the final purpose of sleep, that purpose also obviously must be among the contributory purposes of nocturnal darkness; for that is one of its inevitable and periodical consequences.

The learned and pious Richard Baxter seems to have satisfied himself some centuries ago that sleep was anything but the state of repose which scientists usually assume it to be. In his profound *Inquiry into the Nature of the Soul,* he says:

"The phenomenon of sleep and dreaming, which hath been made use of to exalt the nature of matter, and depress the perfection of the soul; rightly considered shew the very contrary.

"The opposition of appearances observable in this state (of *fatigue* and *activity,* of *insensibility* and *life* at the same time) cannot fail to shew us the opposite natures of the two constituent parts of our composition. If all had been a *blank* of thought and consciousness in sleep, the *soul* would have seemed to be of the same nature with the body: if there had been no *difference* of thought and consciousness *then* and at other times, the *body* would have appeared to be of the same nature with the soul; nor could the *thinking* principle have been so distinguishable.—Who that is rational would choose to be without these informations of an after-existence?—The body no sooner sinks down in weariness and slumber, than this thing within enters fresh upon other scenes of action:—and this without the subserviency of its organs, which are then disabled from its functions. From which it appears, it can be otherwise applied to than by external objects through the senses. Now here is such a *contrariety* of natures obviously discoverable, that it is a wonder men could ever find in their hearts to ascribe them to the same thing."

The marvellous changes wrought in our condition, as well morally as physically, that immediately follow a satisfactory night's rest—changes in no respect less marvellous than those which at shut of day temporarily interrupt our communion with the phenomenal world—require an explanation which the popular notion of sleep does not give. "The morning hour," says a German proverb, "has gold in its mouth." If our sleep has been unimpaired by indiscreet indulgence of the appetites or passions, by unwonted anxieties or otherwise, we awake refreshed, with our strength renewed, our minds serene and clear, our passions calmed, our animosities soothed, with kindlier feelings towards our neighbors than at any other hour of the day. It is the hour, too, which from time immemorial has been consecrated by saint and savage to devotional exercises.

Was it not wisely said by the Rev. Horace Bushnell that "The night is the judgment-bar of the day. About all the reflection there is in the world is due, if not directly to the night, to the habits prepared and fashioned by it"?

"Every one knows," says one of the profoundest living interpreters of the phenomena of life,* "how sweet is the restoration derived from one's pillow in health; more wonderful even yet is that which we derive when sleep occurs at the crisis of severe disease. The nocturnal refreshment of the physical frame induces a similar restoration of the spiritual. Relaxed from the tension in which it is held towards the outer world while awake, during sleep the mind sinks into a condition comparable to that in which it lay before consciousness commenced; all images and shapes it is cognizant of by day either vanish or appear only as reflected pictures; unexcited from without, it gathers itself up into new force, new comprehension of its purpose; much that crossed the waking thoughts, scattered and entangled, becoming thereby sifted and arranged. Hence it is that our waking thoughts are often our truest

* *Life: Its Nature, Varieties, and Phenomena*, by Leo H. Grindon, Lecturer on Botany at the Royal School of Medicine, Manchester. Sixth American edition. J. B. Lippincott Co., Philadelphia, 1892, p. 349.

and finest; and that dreams are sometimes eminent and wise; phenomena incompatible with the idea that we lie down like grass into our organic roots at night and are merely resuscitated as from a winter when we wake. *Man is captured in sleep, not by death, but by his better nature;* to-day runs in through a deeper day to become the parent of to-morrow, and to issue every morning, bright as the morning of life, and of life-size, from the peaceful womb of the cerebellum."

Why should our minds be so much more alert in the morning, and problems which puzzled and defied solution at night be solved without a struggle? Why should lessons we tried in vain to memorize in the evening come to us when we awake, with verbal accuracy?—a common experience with school-children. So things we search for in vain at even-tide we will often know exactly where to look for after a night's sleep. It is then, too, that we feel the charms of nature most keenly; that we are most disposed to extenuate the misconduct of friends and neighbors. In fact, there seems to be an extraordinary welling-up of charity in us during the hours consecrated to what Hesiod, the Greek poet, describes as the Brother of Death and Son of Night.

If, on the other hand, we are suddenly aroused from profound sleep, we are apt for a time to have a dazed feeling, not knowing exactly where we are or the precise import of what is said to us.

We act as though suddenly brought from more congenial and altogether different surroundings, from which we have been wrested reluctantly. Children are apt to cry; adults to scold. We are made happy if permitted to close our eyes again and return whence we came; to the company we had left.

"A man must be next to a devil," said the Rev. Horace Bushnell, "who wakes angry. After his unconscious Sabbath he begins another day, and every day is Monday. How beautifully thus we are drawn, by this kind economy of sleep, to the exercise of all good dispositions! The acrid and sour ingredients of evil, the grudges, the wounds of feeling, the hypochondriac suspicions, the black torments of misanthropy, the morose fault-findings, are so far tempered and sweetened by God's gentle discipline of sleep that we probably do not even conceive how demoniacally bitter they would be if no such kind interruptions broke their spell. . . . Sleep is the perfectly passive side of our existence, and best prepares us to the sense of whatever is to be got by mere receptivity."

Every parent is familiar with the smile that at times comes over a sleeping infant's face, betraying as distinctly as ever when awake its experience of pleasing emotions. The elder Pliny takes note of the occasional habit of infants sucking in their sleep; and also of their sometimes awaking suddenly with every symptom of terror and distress. Lucretius, in the noblest epic poem of the Latin tongue, speaks of race-horses, while sleeping, becoming suddenly bathed in perspiration, breathing heavily, and their muscles strained as if starting in a race; also of the hunting-dogs while fast asleep moving their limbs and yelping as if in pursuit of the deer, until, awaking, they are sadly disabused of their delusions:

"Donec discussis redeant erroribus ad se."*

Bryant concludes "The Land of Dreams," of

*"But more, what Studies please, what most delight,
And fill Mens thoughts, they dream them o're at Night;
The Lawyers plead, make Laws, the Souldiers fight;
The Merchants dream of storms, they hear them roar,
And often shipwrecks leap, or swim to shore:
I think of Natur's powers, my Mind pursues
Her Works, and e'en in Sleep invokes a Muse:
And other Studies too, which entertain
Mens waking thoughts, they dream them o're again.
. . . .
"And not in thoughtful Man alone, but Beast!
For often, sleeping Racers pant and sweat,
Breath short, as if they ran their second Heat;
As if the Barrier down, with eager pace
They strecht, as when contending for the Race.
And often Hounds, when Sleep hath closed their Eyes,
They toss, and tumble, and attempt to rise:
They open often, often snuff the Air,
As if they presst the footsteps of the Deer;
And sometimes wak't pursue their fancy'd prey,
The fancy'd Deer, that seems to run away,
Till quite awak't, the follow'd Shapes decay.
And softer Curs, that lie and sleep at home,
Do often rouse, and walk about the Room,
And bark, as if they saw some Strangers come."
—*De Rerum Natura*, book iv.

which his sleeping daughter Julia is the heroine, with these striking lines:

"Dear maid, in thy girlhood's opening flower,
Scarce weaned from the love of childish play!
The tears on whose cheeks are but the shower
That freshens the blooms of early May!

"Thine eyes are closed, and over thy brow
Pass thoughtful shadows and joyous gleams,
And I know, by thy moving lips, that now
Thy spirit strays in the Land of Dreams.

"Light-hearted maiden, oh, heed thy feet!
Oh, keep where that beam of Paradise falls:
And only wander where thou mayst meet
The blessed ones from its shining walls!

"So shalt thou come from the Land of Dreams,
With love and peace to this world of strife:
And the light which over that border streams
Shall lie on the path of thy daily life."

Another poet of promise, Mr. Watson, has more recently given expression to the same thought in some classical lines, "To the Unknown God":

"When, overarched by gorgeous Night,
I wave my trivial self away;
When all I was to all men's sight
Shares the erasure of the day;
Then do I cast my cumbering load,
Then do I gain a sense of God."

Voltaire tells us that in one of his dreams he

supped with M. Touron, who made the words and music for some verses which he sang. Voltaire in his dream also made some rhymes which he gives:

> "Mon cher Touron, que tu m'enchantes
> Par la douceur de tes accents.
> Que tes vers sont doux et coulants.
> Tu les fais comme tu les chantes."

"In another dream," he adds, "I recited the first canto of the 'Henriade,' but differently from the text. Yesterday I dreamed that verses were recited at supper. Some one remarked that they were too clever—*qu'il y avait trop d'esprit.* I replied that the verses were a fête given to the soul, and ornaments were required for fêtes. Thus I have in my dreams said things that I would hardly have said when awake; I have had reflections in spite of myself, in which I had no part. I had neither will nor freedom, and yet I combined ideas with sagacity, and even with some genius. What then am I if not a machine?"*

In the same paper Voltaire made this important statement: "Whatever theory you adopt, whatever vain efforts you make to prove that your memory moves your brain, and that your brain moves your soul, you are obliged to admit that all your ideas come to you, in sleep, independently of you and in spite of you—your will has no part

* *Dictionnaire Philosophique,* tit. "Somnambuler et Songer."

in them whatever. It is certain, then, that *you may think seven or eight hours consecutively, without having the least desire to think, without even being aware that you think.*"

We read of a monk who had been appointed to write an epitaph for the tomb of the Venerable Bede. Being much puzzled for an adjective applicable to Bede, he fell asleep, and in a dream, it is said, was supplied by an angel with the following lines:

> "Hacce jacent fossâ
> Bedæ venerabilis ossa."

It was to this communication from the land of dreams it is owing that, since Bede's death, "venerabilis" has been uniformly treated as a part of his name. This is the only explanation ever given of its selection.

By far the most voluminous and, after the Bible, the most instructive repository of facts relating to the mysteries of sleep in any literature will be found in the writings of Emanuel Swedenborg, the most illustrious of the Swedish race, especially in the records which he made subsequent to the year 1747, when, as he claimed, his spiritual vision was opened. Of the nature of this illumination it will be sufficient to cite the following passage from a letter which he wrote to the King of Sweden in consequence of the seizure and suppression of some copies of a treatise he had written on Conjugial Love:

" I have already informed your Majesty, and beseech you to recall it to mind, that the Lord our Saviour manifested Himself to me in a sensible personal appearance; that He has commanded me to write what has been already done, and what I have still to do: that He was afterwards graciously pleased to endow me with the privilege of conversing with Angels and Spirits, and to be in fellowship with them. I have already declared this more than once to your Majesties in the presence of all the Royal Family when they were graciously pleased to invite me to their table with five Senators, and several other persons; this was the only subject discoursed of during the repast. Of this I also spoke afterwards to several other Senators; and more openly to their Excellencies Count de Teffein, Count Bonde, and Count Hopken, who are still alive, and who were satisfied with the truth of it. I have declared the same in England, Holland, Germany, Denmark, Spain, and at Paris, to Kings, Princes, and other particular persons, as well as to those in this kingdom. If the common report is believed, the Chancellor has declared, that what I have been reciting are untruths, although the very truth. To say that they cannot believe and give credit to such things, therein will I excuse them, for it is not in my power to place others in the same state that God has placed me, so as to be able to convince them by their own eyes and ears of the truth of those deeds and things I have made publicly known. I have no ability to capacitate them to converse with Angels and Spirits, neither to work miracles to dispose or force their understandings, to comprehend what I say. When my writings are read with attention and cool reflection (in which many things are to be met with as hitherto unknown), it is easy enough to conclude, that I could not come by such knowledge, but by a real vision, and converse with those who are in the Spiritual World. As a further proof, I beseech their Excellencies to peruse what is contained in my Treatise on Conjugial Love, *page 314 to 316.* This book is in the hands of Count D'Ekleblad, and Count de Bjelke. If any doubt shall still remain, I am ready to testify with the most solemn oath that can be offered in this matter, that I have said nothing but essential and real Truth, without any mixture of deception. This knowledge is given to me from our Saviour, not for any particular merit of mine, but for the great concern of all Christians' Salvation and Happiness; and as such, how can any venture to assert it as false? That these things may appear such as many have had no Conception of, and of consequence, that they cannot from thence credit, has nothing remarkable in it, for scarce any thing is known respecting them."

In a letter to Mr. Ostinger, Swedenborg says further:

" To your Interrogation, if there is occasion for any Signs of an Extraordinary Kind to confirm Mankind that I am sent from the Lord to do what I do? I have in reply to observe, that at this day no Signs or Miracles will be given, because they operate only to an outward dead belief, and do not avail so as to convince the Inward State of the mind agreeable to the State of Free-Will given to Man by the Lord, as the proper means of his Regeneration. That miracles only operate to an Exterior Faith or Belief, may be seen from the little effect they had on the people in Egypt, and the Children of Israel in the Desert, when the Lord Jehovah descended on Mount Sinai in their presence: and from what effect they had on the Jewish Nation, when they saw all the miracles our Saviour performed before them; for after all, did they not crucify him at last? So if the Lord was to appear now in the sky, attended with Angels and Trumpets, it would have no other effect than it had then. See Luke xvi. 29, 30, 31. The Signs that will be given at this day, will be an Illumination of the mind from the flowing Graces and Knowledge of the Lord, together with the reception of the Truths of the New Church, which will form the mind to a just perception of Heavenly Truth, that will work more effectually than any Miracles.

"You ask me, if I have spoke with the Apostles? To which I reply, I have. I have spoken at times, during the space of one whole year with Paul, and particularly of what is mentioned in the Epistle to the Romans, chap. iii. 28. I have moreover spoken three times with John; once with Moses; and I suppose a hundred times with Luther, who owned to me that, contrary to the advice and warning of an Angel, he had received the Doctrine of Salvation by Faith alone, merely by itself, and that with the intent that he might make an entire separation from Popery. But with the Angelic Order I have spoke and conversed for these twenty-two years past, and daily continue to converse with them, they being sent of the Lord as Associates. There was no occasion to mention this in my Writings; for had I done it, who would have believed it? Would they not also have said, Do Miracles first, and then we will believe?"

We have English translations of thirty-three substantial octavo volumes, consisting pretty exclusively of what Swedenborg saw or heard in the spiritual world while either asleep or in a state of practically suspended consciousness of the phenomenal world. Irrespective of the theological doctrines developed in most of these volumes, it is impossible to overrate their importance in enlightening us in regard to what goes on in our states of suspended consciousness, and above all, its conclusiveness against any theory of mental or spiritual inactivity while in that condition.

That Swedenborg was as credible a witness of what he believed he heard and saw in the spiritual world as either of the prophets of the old dispensation or apostles of the new, no one familiar with his life and occupations can seriously doubt. For the edification of such of my readers as may not have the advantage of such familiarity, I take the liberty of referring them to some authorities, to which they will hardly hesitate to defer, so far at least as to recognize the extraordinary activity of Swedenborg's psychical nature during the twenty-eight later years of his life, for the larger part of which time he claimed to be in pretty constant communication with the spiritual world.*

The records of these revelations are so accessible that I will not distend this volume by any analysis of them. To most persons I think I shall convey

* Appendix A.

a sufficiently definite general idea of them for my purpose in referring to them here, by setting forth, as I propose to do in the appendix, Swedenborg's account of interviews in the spiritual world with Luther, Melancthon, and Calvin, which I venture to commend to the attention of my readers.*

In connection with Swedenborg's post-obit view of Calvin it may be instructive to read a few extracts from one of the most recent biographies of the great solifidian theologian :†

> "While a boy at school, intensely devoted to study, he cared little for the pastimes in which his fellow-scholars indulged, he shunned society and was more disposed to censure the frivolities of those around him than to secure the solace of their companionship; severe to others, he was still more so to himself, and his pale face and attenuated frame bore witness at once to the rigor of his abstinence and the ardor with which he prosecuted his studies."

While pursuing the study of law at Orleans the same writer says of him:

> "At all times, indeed, a diligent student, he seems at this time to have been impelled by his zeal beyond those bounds which a wise regard to health would impose. It was his wont, after a frugal supper, to labor till midnight, and in the morning when he awoke he would, before he arose, recall and digest what he had read the previous day, so as to make it thoroughly his

* Appendix B.

† W. Lindsay Alexander, D.D., one of the Bible revisers.

own. 'By these protracted vigils,' says Beza, 'he secured indeed a solid erudition and an excellent memory; but it is probable he at the same time sowed the seeds of that disease which occasioned him various illnesses in after life and at last brought upon him premature death.' (He died in his fifty-fourth year.)"

While settled over a parish in Geneva, where, "besides preaching every day in each alternate week, he taught theology three times in the week, attended weekly meetings of his consistory, read the Scriptures once a week in the congregation, carried on an extensive correspondence upon a multiplicity of subjects, and was engaged repeatedly in controversy with the opponents of his opinions," he writes to a friend:

"I have not time to look out of my house at the blessed sun; and if things continue thus I shall forget what sort of appearance it has. When I have settled my usual business I have so many letters to write, so many questions to answer, that *many a night is spent without any offering of sleep being brought to nature*. . . .

"The incessant and exhausting labors to which Calvin gave himself could not but tell on the strongest constitution: how much more on one so fragile as his. Amid many sufferings, however, and frequent attacks of sickness, he manfully pursued his course for twenty-eight years; nor was it till his frail body, torn by many and painful diseases — fever, asthma, stone, and gout —the fruits, for the most part, of his sedentary habits and unceasing activity—had, as it were, fallen to pieces around him — that his indomitable spirit relinquished the conflict. . . . After he had retired from public labors he lingered for some months enduring the severest agony without a murmur and cheerfully attending to all the duties of a private kind which his disease left him strength to discharge."

How different might have been the history of Protestantism in the world had Calvin given as many hours to sleep as he did to professional work, is a problem upon which some reflection would not be wasted by any of us.

CHAPTER IV

Most conspicuous changes wrought during sleep psychical, not physical—Seclusion from the world most perfect in sleep — Why the aged sleep less than others—Mysterious effects of sleep upon the demands of our appetites—Our greater endurance while sleeping than when awake—The need for sleep diminishes as the organization of our lives becomes more complex—Buffon—Æsculapius—Letter of Iamblichus—Mohammed—Cicero's dream.

OF the changes which distinguish our condition in the morning from our condition in the evening, the most conspicuous are not physical, but psychical. The moral side of our being seems for the time to have been in the ascendant. Having ceased for some hours to be preoccupied with what is purely personal, narrow, and narrowing, the world's hold upon our thoughts and affections having been temporarily broken, we seem to have been at liberty for a time to realize that we are a substantive part of the universal life; to feel the spirit of the ages of which we are a product; to look up from nature to nature's God, its author, and to his great world as a manifestation of Him rather than a product of human ingenuity and pretension; all this undisturbed by the calculations and ambitions of our day-lit life.

It was thus "to overcome the world," or at least to assist us in it, that the Mosaic law set apart one day in seven for our spiritual refection, *and enjoined upon us to do no manner of work.* It was for the like purpose we were directed, when we pray, to enter into our inner chamber and shut our door, that we be not distracted by what the world may think or say or be to us while we commune with our Father in heaven. May we not—do we not have a more perfect seclusion from the world in our sleep, to help us to such a direct, prolonged, and undisturbed communion than is possible at any other time? Is it not necessary for all of us, or at least for much the larger proportion of the world who otherwise might never seek this closer communion with God, to be subjected to the operation of a law which for a portion of every day reduces them to a condition in which nothing operates to prevent their giving their attention to the divine messengers that are continually struggling for an opportunity to be heard? This idea appears to have been the happy inspiration of one of our as yet unpublished poets in the following sonnet:

"If thou wouldst look life's problem in the face,
And comprehend her mystic countenance,
Seek, in the early morn, ere yet the grace
Of dewdrops has been withered by the sun,

Some solitary glen or truant brook,
And scan, freed from results of yesterday,
The ill-deciphered pages of life's book:
And ere to-day's vicissitudes have cast
Their shadows o'er the judgment, thou shalt see
Thy blessings will confront thee then, and ask
A recognizing smile. The world shall seem
A higher fact,—the heart of man more wise,
The very universe on larger plan,—
The glamour of day-dawn within thine eyes."*

The changes wrought in us while sleeping, as a rule, vary according to the amount of sleep we require, and that varies with our age. In our childhood we require far more sleep than at later periods of life, and the younger we are, the more we need. Infants, in whom we are able to discern few, if any, traces of a moral sense, sleep most of the time. It is during this period, before their rationality is developed, and before they come under the influence of the world and its temptations, which are so necessary to our spiritual growth later in life—in other words, before the moral sense can be successfully appealed to, that the seed is planted by parental love, which is destined to grow and shelter them from those temptations when they shall assail. The longer hours which infancy requires for sleep are proportioned to their greater spiritual needs. An infant would perish in a few hours if allowed no more sleep than would suffice for an adult.

* Mrs. J. Kennedy Potter.

Old people, whose ties to the world not already severed are daily weakening, spend fewer hours in sleep, as a rule, than the younger of any age.

Why these discriminations of nature between the old, the middle-aged, and the infant? It is not casual, but uniform and universal. Did fatigue create a need for repose, why should the octogenarian, trembling with weakness, sleep least? Why should the infant, who does nothing to induce fatigue, and doubles its weight out of its overflowing abundance of life, in a few months, sleep many times as much as its grandparents? Obviously because we tend to become less active and more contemplative in our declining years. The world has been gradually losing its charm, its former allurements cease to distract; the mind feeds upon the spiritual experiences of a long life, less disturbed than during our earlier years by the temptations of the world, the flesh, and the devil. They therefore may be presumed to need less sleep or to be in a spiritual condition to profit less for any moral purpose by sleep than either the stalwart adult or the puling infant. In the inspired language of the poet Waller,

"The soul's dark cottage, battered and decayed,
Lets in the light through chinks that Time has made."

Following this line of thought, we should pause to take note of the fact that one by one the several senses by which we hold communion with the visible world cease to render their wonted service as we advance into the autumn of life. The eyes, to use Milton's expression, "their seeing have forgot," the ears their hearing, the skin its sensibility, and so on. Why, except that the messages which it is the function of the senses to bring to us from the external world are becoming less needful to us or more hurtful, or that the interruption of those messages is required to supplement the educational offices for which the hours of sleep, usual at that age, were inadequate? With some the senses are dulled earlier than with others. May not this impairment of sensibility reflect a corresponding spiritual or moral condition? Of course, this impairment is a result, not a final cause or purpose. Of what is it so likely to be the result as of a divine purpose, similar to that we are ascribing to sleep, of diminishing or checking the interference of the phenomenal world with our spiritual growth, and an aid to us in overcoming the world, or, rather, our sense of our personal importance to the world?

Rest implies inactivity, a suspension of effort and exertion, the substitution of idleness for labor. If, therefore, all our nobler faculties have been resting during the night, have been doing nothing, by the operation of what force or by what necromancy are we so transfigured in the morning?

The effect of sleep upon the demands of our stomach is also mysterious. Few people take less than three meals daily, if they can help it, yet a man may sleep from twelve to fifteen hours —cases are recorded of persons sleeping much longer—without waking, and of course without taking any nourishment whatsoever.

Wraxall, in his Memoirs, tells us that William Pitt, the most eminent minister of George III. of England, having been much disturbed by a variety of painful political occurrences, "drove out to pass the night with Dundas at Wimbledon. After supper the minister withdrew to his chamber, having given his servant directions to call him at seven on the ensuing morning. No sooner had Pitt retired than Dundas, conscious how much the minister stood in need of repose, repaired to his apartment, locked the door, and put the key in his pocket, at the same time enjoining the valet on no consideration to disturb his master, but to allow him to sleep as long as nature required. It is a truth that Pitt neither awoke nor called any person till half-past four in the afternoon of the following day, when Dundas, entering his room together with his servant, found him still in so deep a sleep that it became necessary to shake in order to awaken him. He had slept uninterruptedly during more than sixteen hours."

Such long naps, we fancy, are by no means uncommon, but are not heard of—like the heroes before Agamemnon—*carent quia vate sacro.*

It is reported of Lord Brougham that when he returned home after his brilliant and exhausting defence of Queen Caroline he went at once to bed, with orders not to be disturbed, however long he might sleep — orders which his household obeyed, though with astonishment deepening into something like terror as the young lawyer's nap prolonged itself for nearly eight-and-forty hours. His physician afterwards declared that this sleep had saved him from brain fever, though probably only the marvellously recuperative powers which he possessed enabled him to take nature's remedy in one such mighty dose.

Yet all this time the digestion and other functions of the body have been going on very much as they are wont during the waking hours. It thus appears that we require nourishment three or four times more frequently while awake than while sleeping. Yet—and here is another surprise—we usually awake in the morning without either hunger or faintness, one or the other of which always accompanies an unusually long fast when awake. The first and morning meal is ordinarily the lightest of the day among people who are free to consult their tastes about their hours for eating. How shall we explain this strange discrepancy in the actions of the stomach in the daytime and at night? It is no answer to say that we work in the daytime, hence waste and hunger; for the same necessity for frequent nourishment during the day is as surely experienced by a person taking little or no physical exercise as by the bricklayer or the wood-sawyer. Obviously a condition of things has been superinduced by sleep which involves not only a discontinuance of intercourse with the phenomenal world, but a suspension of some of its sternest exactions.

There is another extraordinary result of sleep which, so far as I know, has never been remarked upon, but which accredits, if it does not explain, some of the stories related in the Bible which put our faith in the divine origin of that record to the severest test.

When one lays himself down upon his bed or couch, however tired, if awake, he rarely remains long in any one position. At frequent intervals he feels an impulse to turn over or move some of his limbs, or otherwise relieve himself from what has become an uncomfortable position.

If he falls asleep, however, though he has the ground for a bed and a log or even a stone for a pillow, he may lie quietly for many hours without the slightest motion of any kind save that incident to involuntary respiration. Nor, when he awakes, will he experience any discomfort in any part of his body, not even in that which has sustained the most pressure — a pressure which while awake he would not contentedly have quietly endured for five minutes.

Whence this difference? There is no change in the physical condition of the sleeper that will account for it. His body weighs no less, the blood circulates as freely in the veins, and when he awakes, as a rule, he not only may have no sense of pain or discomfort anywhere, but, on the contrary, feel refreshed at every point. What has occasioned this mysterious change in the relations of causes and effects on a sleeping from those operations on a waking man?

We are told that Jacob, the son of Isaac and grandson of Abraham, on his journey towards Padan Aram in quest of a wife, "lighted upon a certain place and tarried there all night, because the sun was set." (We are not told that he was even tired.) "And he took one of the stones of the place and put it under his head and lay down in that place to sleep." In his sleep the young man had dreams of an inconceivably glorious future. When he awoke he exclaimed: "Surely the Lord is in this place and I knew it not; this is none other than the house of God and the gate of heaven." He rose, took the stone that he had put under his head and set it up for a pillar and poured oil upon it. And he called the name of that place Bethel.

What change did sleep work in Jacob during that night, with a stone for his pillow, that he should set that stone up for a monument and pour oil upon the top of it and finally make of it the dwelling-place of his God?

The reason assigned in the sacred record is that during his sleep he "beheld a ladder set upon the earth and the top of it reached to heaven, and he beheld angels, the messengers from God, ascending and descending on it, and the Lord standing above it, who, besides promising that Jacob's seed should be as the dust of the earth for multitude, and that in his seed should all the families of the earth be blessed, added, "Behold I am with thee and will keep thee whithersoever thou goest, and will bring thee again unto this land; for I will not leave thee until I have done that which I have spoken to thee of."

No one will pretend that a communication of such incalculable importance would ever be made by any one, least of all by the God of gods, to one whose mind was, like his body, in a deep sleep. Is it not equally clear that the peculiar time for making it was selected because in his waking hours Jacob would not have been in a condition to receive it?

Who shall say that such ladders are or have ever been uncommon means of communication between the inhabitants of the heavens and the earth, and that angels are not frequently ascending and descending them with heavenly messages to unconscious sleepers?

As we descend in the scale of organized life, the proportion of time spent in sleep seems to increase until we reach a point where life is apparently a continuous sleep. "An oyster," says Buffon, "which does not seem to have any sensible exterior movement nor external sense, is a creature formed to sleep always. A vegetable is in this sense but an animal that sleeps, and, in general, the functions of every organized being lacking power of movement and the senses may be compared to the functions of an animal who should be constrained by nature to sleep continually.

"In the animal the state of sleep is not an accidental one, occasioned by the greater or less exercise of its faculties while awake; it is, on the contrary, an essential mode of being, which serves as the base of all animal economy. Our existence begins in sleep; the fœtus sleeps almost continually, and the infant sleeps more hours than it is awake.

"Sleep, which appears to be a purely passive state, a species of death, is, on the contrary, the first state of the living animal and the foundation of life. It is not a privation, an annihilation; it is a mode of being, a style of existence as real and more general than any other. We exist in this state before existing in any other; all organized beings which have not the senses exist in this state only, while none exist in a state of continual movement, and all existences participate more or less in this state of repose."*

As we rise in the scale of organized life, on the other hand, we find that the time required for sleep diminishes, and the quality of life exhibits a corresponding increase of complexity, and a corresponding enlargement of function, until we reach the highest of organizations, our own species.

* "Discours sur la Nature des Animaux." *Œuvres de Buffon.* Édition Flourens, vol. ii. p. 331.

At the close of a laborious day we invariably, if in health, feel a languor which prompts us to take a position in which the weight of our bodies will be so distributed as to invite sleep—for which, if in health, we do not have to wait long. The interval between its arrival and our laying ourselves in a recumbent position is usually one of exquisite pleasure.

All our impressions of sleep are formed before it arrives and after it begins to leave. We enjoy what we call going to sleep, and we enjoy the feelings we experience after we have slept, but during sleep we have no consciousness of any sensation which we have any right to attribute directly and exclusively to it, or of which our senses can take cognizance. While it is thus made pleasant for us to close our eyes and relax our hold upon the world for a portion of every twenty-four hours, we have no more right to infer that it is merely that we may remain in a pleasing state of inactivity and insensibility than we have to infer that the final purpose of hunger is to secure us the gratifications of the palate, or the final purpose of sexual attraction is merely to gratify our sensuality. As in both these cases, the ends to be reached are of the most far-reaching character, and the desires are given that the means for the accomplishment of those ends should not be neglected, so our diurnal desire for sleep is manifestly designed to promote in us the growth and development of spiritual graces in some way, for which the waking hours are less propitious. Our Maker could have had no other design in our creation; He can have no other design in the perpetuation of our race. Why should Infinite Wisdom have assigned a less important function for the very considerable portion of our lives during which our consciousness is suspended in sleep than to the function of hunger or lust? Why should we resist the obvious implication that in falling asleep we are being gradually separated from the world of the senses, and, as they seem to recede, that something flows into us which yields a pleasure that grows more unmixed and absolute until consciousness of our external and natural life altogether ceases?

" As angels in some brighter dreams
Call to the soul when man doth sleep;
So some strange thoughts transcend our wonted themes
And into glory peep."

Pausanias, in his historic tour in Greece, describes a temple erected in honor of Æsculapius, in the court of which he found the figure of Oneiros, the god of dreams, and beside it another of Hypnos, or Sleep, putting a lion to sleep. To this latter figure, says Pausanias, they had given the name of Epidotes, or the Giver.*

" So He giveth his beloved in their sleep."

* From the Greek word ἐπιδίδωμι, to increase, to fatten, to give freely, to give as a benevolence.

From the writings of Iamblichus, at one time the head of the school of Neo-Platonists, it appears that the view here taken of sleep, as having a higher function than simply the reparation of waste, was shared some fifteen centuries ago by thoughtful men, who did not claim to speak by divine inspiration. In a letter compiled from his writings, and quoted by R. A. Vaughan in his *Hours with the Mystics*, he says:

" There is nothing unworthy of belief in what you have been told concerning the sacred sleep and divination by dreams. I explain it thus:

" The soul has a twofold life, a lower and a higher. In sleep the soul is freed from the constraint of the body, and enters, as one emancipated, on its divine life of intelligence. Then, as the noble faculty which beholds the objects that truly are the objects in the world of intelligence stirs within and awakens to its power, who can be surprised that the mind, which contains in itself the principles of all that happens, should, in this, the state of liberation, discern the future in those antecedent principles which will make that future what it is to be? *The nobler part of the soul is thus united by abstraction to higher natures, and becomes a participant in the wisdom and foreknowledge of the gods.*

" Recorded examples of this are numerous and well authenticated; instances occur, too, every day. Numbers of sick, by sleeping in the temple of Æsculapius, have had their cure revealed to them in dreams vouchsafed by the god. Would not Alexander's army have perished but for a dream, in which Dionysius pointed out the means of safety? Was not the siege of Aphritis raised through a dream sent by Jupiter Ammon to Lysander? *The night-time of the body is the daytime of the soul.*"

Tradition accounts for Mohammed's being among the prophets in this wise: While indulging in spiritual meditations and repeating pious exercises on Mount Hira in the month of Ramedan, the Angel Gabriel came to him by night, *as he was sleeping,* held a silken scroll before him, and required him, though not knowing how to read, to recite what was written on the scroll. The words thus communicated remained graven on his memory, and ran as follows:

> "Read! In the name of the Lord who created man from a drop. Read! For the Lord is the Most High, who hath taught by the pen to man what he knew not. Nay truly, man walketh in delusion when he deems that he suffices for himself. To thy Lord they must all return."

This brief announcement of the Angel Gabriel to Mohammed in his sleep deserves to be regarded as the corner-stone of the religion of the most numerous of the monotheistic sects in the world to this day—a religion which Napoleon I. characteristically pronounced superior to Christianity in that it conquered half the world in ten years, while Christianity took three hundred years to establish itself.

Cicero tells us of a dream he had of a singularly prophetic character which occurred to him in one of the stages of his flight after his banishment from Rome. He is certainly a good witness, and his dream cannot easily be reconciled with the popular notion of mental and moral inactivity during sleep.

Being lodged in the villa of a friend, after he had lain restless and wakeful a great part of the night, he fell into a sound sleep near break of day, and when he waked, about eight in the morning, told his dream to those round him: That as he seemed to be wandering disconsolate in a lonely place, Caius Marius, with his fasces wreathed with laurel, accosted him, and demanded why he was so melancholy; and when he answered that he was driven out of his country by violence, Marius took him by the hand, and, bidding him be of courage, ordered the next lictor to conduct him into his monument, telling him that there he should find safety. Upon this the company presently cried out that he would have a quick and glorious return. All of which was exactly fulfilled; for his restoration was decreed in a certain temple built by Marius, and, for that reason, called Marius's Monument, where the Senate happened to be assembled on that occasion.

CHAPTER V

The most important events in human history initiated during sleep—Altruism first taught in sleep—Extraordinary spiritual uses of sleep recorded in the Bible.

THE most considerable and imposing repository of facts from which we are authorized to infer anything of what may be going on in us while we sleep may be found where, ordinarily, one would be least likely to look for it, and if sleep be, as most people suppose, simply an interruption of activities for the purpose of repose and refreshment, where it would be most out of place—that is, in the sacred Scriptures. If these writings are what they purport to be—an inspired guide to assist man in leading a holy life—it is impossible to reconcile the prominence they give to the phenomena of sleep with the idea of its being merely a mode of rest from fatigue.

Even a hasty reference to its pages will satisfy the reader that sleep is rarely referred to in the Bible except with reference to some of the most vital processes of spiritual growth or degeneration. In reading the illustrations of this statement, to some of which I will now refer, the reader is requested to note the incalculably important consequences of which, in each case, sleep is the prelude.

In the Bible the very first allusion to sleep associates it with an event second in importance, perhaps, to no other in the history of our race:

> " And the Lord God caused a deep sleep to fall upon the Man, and he slept; and he took one of his ribs, and closed up the flesh instead thereof: and the rib, which the Lord God had taken from the man, made he a woman, and brought her unto the man. And the man said, This is now bone of my bone, and flesh of my flesh: she shall be called Woman, because she was taken out of man. *Therefore shall a man leave his father and his mother, and shall cleave unto his wife: and they shall be one flesh.*"*

Thus it was during his sleep that man was first qualified to love something *outside of himself,* that our race received its first lesson in altruism; experienced its first triumph over the tyranny of its selfhood, and that the institution of matrimony was established. His Eve is man's first unselfish love—his first genuine charity.

Whether regarded as literal or symbolical, the passage quoted is no less impressive and significant.

It was when the sun was going down and a deep sleep fell upon Abram, that the Lord made him the founder of nations; commissioned him

* Genesis ii. 21.

to teach to a pagan world the unity of the God-head and the errors of polytheism.*

It was when Jacob was sent to his grandfather to seek a wife among the daughters of his uncle Laban that he had the dream already referred to, when he beheld a ladder set up on the earth and reaching to heaven, on which the angels of God were ascending and descending, and when he was promised that his seed should be as the dust of the earth and in it all the families of the earth should be blessed.

One of the most pathetic and dramatic stories in all literature is that of Jacob's son, Joseph, and his brethren, the machinery of which consists mainly of dreams. It was the recital of one of *his dreams* that provoked his brethren to sell him into Egypt. While in prison, in consequence of a malicious accusation of his master's wife, he interprets correctly the dreams of the king's chief butler and chief baker, who were his fellow-prisoners. The fame of this achievement spread through the land, and when Pharaoh, the king, was himself perplexed *by a dream,* he sent for Joseph, and was so impressed with his skill in interpreting it that he at once gave him power second only to his own in the kingdom; made him lord of all his house, and ruler over all the land of Egypt. It was thus through dreams that he was enabled to save his brethren "alive

* Genesis xv. 12.

by a great deliverance," to prepare the way for the escape of the children of Israel from the bondage of spiritual darkness in Egypt, to wander forty years in the wilderness, that they might be fitted for a home in a land flowing with milk and honey, and symbolize for all future time the several stages of man's spiritual regeneration.

When Miriam and Aaron railed against Moses for marrying a Cushite woman and said, "Hath the Lord spoken only with Moses; hath he not spoken also with us?" the Lord came down in a pillar of cloud, called Miriam and Aaron before Him, and said: "If there be a prophet among you, I, the Lord, will make myself known unto him *in a vision;* I will speak with him *in a dream.* My servant Moses is not such; he is faithful in all mine house; with him will I speak, mouth to mouth, even manifestly and not in dark speeches; and the form of the Lord shall he behold; wherefore then were ye not afraid to speak against my servant, against Moses?"*

Samuel was laid down to sleep in the temple of the Lord where the ark of God was when the Lord called him by name. "Now Samuel did not yet know the Lord, neither was the word of the Lord yet revealed to him." The Lord called him three times before he knew who it was that called, and then only at the suggestion of the high-priest he answered, "Speak, for thy servant

* Numbers xii. 2–8.

heareth. The Lord then said to Samuel, Behold I will do a thing in Israel at which both the ears of every one that heareth it shall tingle." At the close of the Lord's statement of what He proposed to do, it is recorded that "Samuel grew, and the Lord was with him, and did let none of his words fall to the ground."* "And all Israel from Dan even to Beersheba knew that Samuel was established to be a prophet of the Lord."†

Saul was asleep in his camp when Abishai said to David, whom Saul was pursuing: "God hath delivered up thine enemy into thine hand this day: now therefore let me smite him, I pray thee, with the spear to the earth at one stroke, and I will not smite him the second time." David replied, "The Lord forbid that I should put forth mine hand against the Lord's anointed."

When Saul awoke on hearing the voice of David from a neighboring hill, whither he had taken refuge, reproaching Abner for not having kept better watch over the Lord's anointed, he said: "I have sinned: return, my son David: for I will no more do thee harm, because my life was precious in thine eyes this day: behold, I have played the fool, and have erred exceedingly. . . . Blessed be thou, my son David: thou shalt both do mightily, and shalt surely prevail."‡

To King Solomon is attributed the memorable 127th Psalm, in which occur the following lines:

* 1 Samuel iii. 19. † *Ib.* iii. 20. ‡ *Ib.* xxvi. 21, 25.

"Except the Lord build the house,
They labor in vain that build it:
Except the Lord keep the city,
The watchman waketh but in vain.
It is vain for you that ye rise up early, and so late
take rest,
And eat the bread of toil:
For so he giveth unto his beloved in their sleep."

Among the proverbs of the same king, the most famous of all earthly kings for his wisdom, "sweet sleep" is held forth as one of the privileges of him who despiseth not "the chastenings of the Lord" nor is "weary of his reproof." *

While Daniel and his three comrades were living at the court of Nebuchadnezzar, "God gave them knowledge and skill in all learning and wisdom: and Daniel had understanding in all visions and dreams."

When two years later Nebuchadnezzar had a dream which he had forgotten, he issued a decree for the slaughter of all his wise men and magicians, because they could not make known to him the dream and its interpretation. Daniel saved their lives and his own by revealing to the king "the visions of his head upon his bed," and their interpretation. One of the memorable results of this dream was that Nebuchadnezzar at last confessed to Daniel that his God was the God of gods and the Lord of kings, and he made

* Proverbs iii. 11.

Daniel himself to rule over the whole province of Babylon and to be chief governor over all the wise men of Babylon.*

Nebuchadnezzar in due time had another dream, which Daniel was called upon to interpret. It was of painful import. The king was to be driven from men; his dwelling was to be with the beasts of the field; he was to be made to eat grass as oxen and to be wet with the dew of heaven, and seven times were to pass over him until he should know "the Most High ruleth in the kingdom of men and giveth it to whomsoever he will." "At the end of the days," said Nebuchadnezzar in his official proclamation of this experience, "I lifted up mine eyes unto heaven, and . . . at the same time mine understanding returned unto me; and for the glory of my kingdom, my majesty and brightness returned unto me; . . . and I was established in my kingdom, and excellent greatness was added unto me. Now I Nebuchadnezzar praise and extol and honor the King of heaven; for all his works are truth, and his ways judgment: and those that walk in pride he is able to abase."†

The prophet Joel, speaking in the name of the Lord God, gives us very distinctly to understand that it is in the visions of the night that God pours out his spirit upon us: "It shall come to pass afterward, that I will pour out my spirit

* Daniel ii. 47. † *Ib.* iv. 5.

upon all flesh; and your sons and your daughters shall prophesy, your old men shall dream dreams, your young men shall see visions: and also upon the servants and upon the handmaids in those days will I pour out my spirit."*

The angel of God spake unto Jacob in a dream, saying: "Lift up now thine eyes, and see that all the rams which leap upon the cattle are speckled, ringstreaked, and grizzled: for I have seen all that Laban doeth unto thee." "Now arise, get thee out from this land, and return unto the land of thy kindred."

Thereupon Jacob, with Rachel his wife, and Leah, stole away with their children, their cattle, and their goods, unawares to Laban the Syrian. The third day after Jacob's flight Laban first heard of it, and after a seven days' journey overtook him in the Mount Gilead.

Meantime, *God came to Laban the Syrian in a dream by night,* and said unto him, "Take heed that thou speak not to Jacob either good or bad." When Laban met Jacob he chided him for going away secretly, and said: "It is in the power of my hand to do you hurt: but the God of your father spake unto me yesternight, saying, Take thou heed that thou speak not to Jacob, either good or bad."

It was then and after these three communications from on high that the covenant between

* Joel ii. 28.

Laban and Jacob was entered into at Mispah and they separated in peace.

When Gideon's faith in the Lord's promise to aid him in a war against the Midianites had been miraculously confirmed, we are told that "it came to pass *the same night* that the Lord said unto him, Take thy father's bullock, even the second bullock of seven years old, and throw down the altar of Baal that thy father hath, and cut down the Asherah goddess that is by it, and build an altar unto the Lord thy God upon the top of this stronghold, in the orderly manner, and take the second bullock and offer a burnt offering with the wood of the Asherah which thou shalt cut down."

The same night the Lord directed Gideon to go with his servants and visit the camp of the Midianites, "and when Gideon was come behold there was a man that told a dream unto his fellow and said, Behold I dreamed a dream, and, lo, a cake of barley bread tumbled into the camp of Midian and came unto the tent and smote it that it fell, and turned it upside down that the tent lay along. And his fellow answered and said, This is nothing else save the sword of Gideon, the son of Joash, a man of Israel; into his hand God hath delivered Midian and all the host."

And *the same night* Gideon and his hundred men attacked the Midianites and put them to flight.

It will be observed that each of the three miraculous processes by which the enemies of the true

Church were overcome and dispersed were all performed in the night; and one of them—apparently the most important—was the result of a dream.

When Elijah was a refugee from the persecutions of Jezebel, and, faint with hunger, had fallen *asleep* under a juniper-tree, an angel touched him and told him to "arise and eat."* "He arose, and did eat and drink, and went in the strength of that meat forty days and forty nights unto Horeb, the mount of God."

We read in Job that:

> "By reason of the multitude of oppressions they cry out;
> They cry for help by reason of the arm of the mighty.
> But none saith, Where is God my Maker,
> *Who giveth songs in the night;*
> Who teacheth us more than the beasts of the earth,
> And maketh us wiser than the fowls of the air?"

"I will bless the Lord, who hath given me counsel," says the Royal Psalmist; "my reins also instruct me in the night seasons." †

"Thou hast proved my heart; *thou hast visited me in the night;* thou hast tried me and findest nothing; I am purposed that my mouth shall not transgress." ‡

"Where there is *no vision*," said Solomon, "the people cast off restraint." §

* 1 Kings xix. 5.
† Psalm xvi. 7.
‡ Psalm xvii. 3.
§ Proverbs xxix. 18.

"For the Lord will command his loving kindness in the daytime, and *in the night* his *song shall be with me.*" *

The exclusive use of the hours usually consecrated to sleep to herald the birth of our Saviour is so remarkable that it is impossible for an enlightened Christian to read the story as reported by Matthew without feeling that as He was heralded to his parents and the wise men of the East who were sent to search for Him, He is heralded to all of us in the visions of the night "when God pours out his spirit upon all flesh."

His birth was foretold by an angel of the Lord who appeared unto Joseph in a dream, saying, "Joseph, thou son of David, fear not to take unto thee Mary thy wife: for that which is conceived in her is of the Holy Ghost. And she shall bring forth a Son; and thou shalt call his name Jesus; for it is he that shall save his people from their sins."†

The same event was announced by an angel directly to Mary, though not in her sleep, and that she was to be the mother of our Saviour. The Magnificat which she pronounced when she visited Elizabeth, immediately after the conception, shows how conscious she was of the "day star" that had risen in her heart. Joseph, on the other hand, was minded to put her away privily because he had no comprehension of the

* Psalm xlii. 8. † Matthew i. 20.

significance and import of this new birth. An angel, therefore, was sent to him *in his sleep* "to tell him not to fear to take Mary for his wife," and so Joseph arose from his sleep and did as the angel of the Lord commanded him.

Mary was spiritually prepared for this new birth. Joseph was not. He judged as the world judged; as the Apostles were judged by their hearers, and as Paul was judged by Festus. He had to be taught in his sleep what he might never have received while awake and under worldly influences. The world may be presumed to have had no such hold, then, upon Mary.

The wise men who were sent by Herod to Bethlehem to search out carefully the young child Jesus, and, when found, report the place to him, *were warned in a dream* that they should not return to Herod, so they departed into their own country another way.

When they were departed, an angel of the Lord appeared to Joseph again *in a dream,* saying: "Arise and take the young child and his mother and flee into Egypt."

After the death of Herod an angel of the Lord appeared once more *in a dream* to Joseph in Egypt, saying: "Arise and take the young child and his mother, and go into the land of Israel: for they are dead that sought the young child's life." Hearing, however, that Herod's son was reigning over Judea, he feared to go thither, and *in consequence of being warned of God in a dream,* he withdrew into the parts of Galilee, to a city called Nazareth.

It is to be observed here that everything done to bring about the birth and protection of the infant Jesus was done in obedience to angelic promptings received in visions of the night; but no such promptings were received by Herod or by the magi, whose interests in the birth of Jesus, great as they were, were of a worldly character.

When Jesus took with Him Peter and James and John and went up into the mountain to pray, there talked with Him two men, Moses and Elias, who appeared in glory.

Peter, and they that were with him, were *heavy with sleep, but when they were fully awake they saw his glory.* Peter then said:

> " Master, it is good for us to be here: and let us make three tabernacles; one for thee, and one for Moses, and one for Elijah: not knowing what he said.
>
> " And while he said these things, there came a cloud, and overshadowed them: . . . and a voice came out of the cloud, saying, This is my Son, my chosen: hear ye him. And when the voice came, Jesus was found alone."*

Till then Jesus, Moses, and Elijah, in Peter's mind, were of equal dignity and equally entitled to tabernacles. After receiving the message from the clouds his spiritual eyes were opened to see

* Luke ix. 33.

the difference between Jesus and his companions, and then he saw no one but Jesus.

The last hours of our Saviour on earth were signalized by an incident no less pertinent to this inquiry and no less remarkable than any of those which heralded his birth.

While Pilate was sitting on the judgment-seat at the trial of Jesus he received the following message from his wife:

> "Have thou nothing to do with that righteous man: for I have suffered many things this day in a dream because of him."*

How interesting beyond expression it would be to know the tenor of this noble lady's dream about "that righteous man," an outcast from his own people, whom she had probably never seen, of whom she could have known nothing except from the priests and pharisees who were clamoring for his life; who belonged to a race held in abhorrence by the Roman aristocracy, and about whom she had been warned of things of so grave a nature as to impel her to interrupt the deliberations of the tribunal over which her husband presided, to warn him to assume no responsibility for whatever the Jews under their laws might do with their prisoner. Of that woman—the last of her sex from whom any ex-

* Matthew xxvii. 19.

pression of sympathy for Jesus in his lifetime emanated that has survived Him—we know not even the name; nothing but the memorable message which she sent to her husband.

History for more than twenty centuries has treated Cornelia, the mother of the Gracchi, as the ideal Roman matron, but a greater than Cornelia sent that message to Pilate.

Nor does the significance of that extraordinary dream end here. As we pursue the story of this most famous and important of all judicial proceedings, and when the Jews clamored that Barabbas rather than Jesus should be pardoned, Pilate asks: "What then shall I do with Jesus which is called Christ?" they all said, "Let him be crucified." Finding that a tumult would be the consequence of resisting any longer the passions of the crowd, Pilate "took water and washed his hands before the multitude, saying, 'I am innocent of the blood of *this righteous man:* see ye to it.'"

The character of Jesus which Pilate's wife had learned in her dream and communicated in her message, her husband not only accepts but proclaims from his judgment-seat. This is the first time the righteousness of Jesus was ever proclaimed by any officer of any government of Rome.

While Peter was waiting for his dinner in Joppa he fell into a trance, when he dreamed the heaven opened and a vessel descended wherein were all manner of four-footed beasts and creeping things of the earth and fowls of the heaven. "And there came a voice to him, Rise, Peter, kill and eat. But Peter said, Not so, Lord; for I have never eaten anything that is common and unclean. And a voice came unto him again a second time, What God hath cleansed, make thou not unclean."* While Peter, much perplexed, thought on the vision, the messengers sent by the Lord to bring him to Cornelius, a devout man and one who feared God, arrived. Peter accompanied them to Cornelius, who had called his friends together in the sight of God to hear from Peter all things that the Lord had commanded him.

Why was Peter put in a trance except the better to qualify him to receive the instructions which he afterwards executed, and which he could not have executed without such instructions?

Cornelius was of the Italian band, not a Jew; hence the lesson Peter taught him in the trance, which was—First, to teach, what the Jews did not believe as a rule, or even suspect, that God is no respecter of persons, but that "in every nation he that feareth him and worketh righteousness is acceptable to him." Secondly, to teach that Jesus was ordained of God to be the Judge of the quick and the dead, and that "through his

*Acts x. 9–16.

name every one that believeth on him shall receive remission of sins."

As a result of these teachings we are told that the Holy Ghost fell upon all them that heard Peter, and they were amazed because that on the Gentiles also was poured out the gift of the Holy Ghost, and when Peter returned to Jerusalem, and was called to account for what he had done by them of the circumcision, he explained what he had done and how he came to do it. Thereupon they "held their peace and glorified God, saying, Then to the Gentiles also hath God granted repentance unto life."

No one can fail to see that the character and scope of these lessons were worthy of their divine origin and could have had no other. It is equally apparent that, to impress these lessons upon the children of men, it was necessary that Peter's consciousness and this-worldliness should first be suspended by sleep.

The Apostle Peter was sleeping between two soldiers and bound with two chains, when "an angel of the Lord stood by him, and a light shined in the cell: and he smote Peter on the side, and awoke him, saying, Rise up quickly. And his chains fell off from his hands."

The most definite and explicit statement of what doubtless deserves to be regarded as the ultimate—the vital—purposes of sleep that is given in the Bible will be found in the rebuke administered to Job by Elihu, the youngest of his comforters, for presuming to question the justice of the trials he was enduring.

"Surely," said Elihu, "thou hast spoken in my hearing, and I have heard the voice of thy words, saying, I am clean, without transgression; I am innocent, neither is there iniquity in me: behold, he findeth occasions against me, he counteth me for his enemy; he putteth my feet in the stocks, he marketh all my paths. Behold, I will answer thee; in this thou art not just; for God is greater than man. Why dost thou strive against him? For he giveth not account of any of his matters. For God speaketh once, yea twice, though man regardeth it not. *In a dream, in a vision of night, when deep sleep falleth upon men, in slumberings upon the bed,* THEN HE OPENETH THE EARS OF MEN, AND SEALETH THEIR INSTRUCTION, THAT HE MAY WITHDRAW MAN FROM HIS PURPOSE AND HIDE PRIDE FROM MAN; HE KEEPETH BACK HIS SOUL FROM THE PIT, AND HIS LIFE FROM PERISHING BY THE SWORD." *

Have we not here a plain and unequivocal statement—

First. That the processes of spiritual growth and development are not only not interrupted, but are more than ordinarily active during sleep.

* Job xxxiii. 8–18.

Secondly. That while in that state man is withdrawn from his own purposes for much higher purposes than animate him during his waking hours.

Thirdly. That it is while sleeping God openeth the ears of men and sealeth their instruction, and that, like the children of Israel in their journey through the wilderness, we are guided in the daytime by God's cloud, in the night by his light. Doth not his cloud limit our horizon even while revealing the path we are to take, to hide us from our enemies, while his light by night enlarges our horizon: so that we can see why, as well as where, we are to prosecute our journey?

How could the purposes of sleep be more explicitly stated, assuming the competence of the authority stating them? How could their importance be made more impressive?

What events are recorded in the whole range of secular history, I will not say of graver, but of equal, import to any one of these I have cited, to which sleep is treated as a necessary incident?

There are some who affect to make light of the Bible story. Conceding for a moment that it is a work of the imagination, a tradition, a myth, a literature merely why is the machinery of sleep so constantly introduced on occasions of such incomparable importance? Why were not these several communications, or revelations, made directly to the parties interested in their waking hours? Why were the hours of sleep chosen when only the Divinity could know whether the communications were received and whether the effect intended was to be realized?

Are we not compelled to suppose it was because a divine truth was more sure of receiving attention; was less liable to encounter worldly obstructions and distractions during the sleeping than during the waking hours?

When the Master wishes to address us we may be sure that He will select the moment most favorable to secure our attention. It is not conceivable that He should select any other than the most favorable. And if, not only in these two or three cases, but, I may say, so uniformly throughout the whole history of the Church, He selected the hours when our consciousness was suspended, to influence our will, are we not logically bound to presume that the suspension of our consciousness for certain hours of every day is mainly, if not exclusively, a part of his plan to secure access to our souls without interfering with the freedom of our wills? Is it not in those hours of suspended consciousness that, in his unfailing love and mercy, He adjusts the balance between the forces of good and evil which are always struggling with each other in our souls, during our waking hours at least, like the "two manner of people" in Rebekah's womb; and that, in that way, He defends and protects our power to choose between good and evil, between right and wrong, between righteousness and sin, without which protection no spiritual growth would be possible? For it is only by his providential maintenance of the equilibrium between the forces of good and evil operating upon us in this life that we are enabled, through every stage of spiritual and moral degeneration, to retain the power to pursue the right and eschew the wrong.

Every enlightened Christian understands that we are created and placed in the world for a purpose which contemplates an eternity of existence, during which we are expected to be constantly growing more into the image of our Creator. Is it reasonable or even credible to suppose that one-third, or indeed any minutest portion, of our terrestrial lives would necessarily have to be spent in a state or under conditions in which no progress whatever can be made in spiritual growth—in regenerate life? To entertain such a belief is to question the essential attributes of Divinity. He who grows not in his sleep, says an old Gaelic proverb, will not grow when awake.

Men of science are notoriously agnostics and materialists, and yet they pass their lives trying to learn the laws of the universe, which are the perfect expression of divine order. The more of those laws we know, the more we ought to believe in the Maker of those laws, while the effect upon the scientist seems to be exactly the reverse. "I recognize no distinction between matter and spirit; I know nothing but force," once wrote the late President Walker to me.

CHAPTER VI

Spiritual influence of sleep illustrated by its privation—Diseases resulting—Toussaint L'Ouverture's defence of Hayti—Difference in sleeping habits of domestic and of predatory animals—Low average of longevity among savages explained — Habits of venomous and non-venomous serpents contrasted — Prominence of sleep in the machinery of Shakespeare's plays—Dr. Wilkinson—Marie Manaceine—Byron's *English Bards and Scotch Reviewers*—Alexander von Humboldt.

THUS far we have studied the function of sleep from its effects, and some of its uses. Now let us look a little further into the effect of its privation.

The sick in a high fever get little sleep. In time they are apt to become delirious. If they recover it is almost uniformly after an unusually prolonged and quiet sleep. In their fever and delirium their thought and speech are almost invariably of the world in which they live, its interests and concerns. Wise physicians insist that a patient under treatment should never be awakened even to take medicine. There is no symptom they welcome so cordially in a patient as a natural sleep, and no change from which they expect more favorable results.

The effect of being awakened from a sound sleep is always unpleasant. It is apt to make one unsocial and irritable. Any such abrupt recall to worldly cares induces a feeling of discontent, such as usually accompanies all unwelcome changes of condition or unpleasant interruptions. Nor is it without significance that grown people pretty universally prefer to be left alone for some time after waking, while we rarely find any who have been much immersed in worldly cares whose friends are not content to leave them alone for a time after waking.

It is the struggle we experience in exchanging abruptly the society we may have left in the land of dreams for that which we meet in the forum or on the exchange that has brought some stimulating beverages, such as coffee or tea or beer, into such general use early in the day throughout the world. On waking, and before we experience any appetite for food, we are prone to welcome an exhilarant of some sort to overcome our reluctance to return to the disciplinary life into which we were born to be trained.

The most compact and instructive statement of the physical evils that follow the privation of sleep that has fallen under my eyes will be found in a work entitled *Diseases of Modern Life.* The author, Benjamin Ward Richardson, was for many years, and until his comparatively recent death, one of the leading members of the Royal College of Physicians in London. In the eighteenth chapter of this work, treating of disease from late hours and broken sleep, he says:

"Although it is impossible to define in one term any one disease originating from irregular sleep and late hours of retiring to rest, there are certain impairments resulting from these habits which influence the course of the health and help materially to shorten life. . . .

"If, in the period of his early life, a man breaks the rule against nature and by a strong and persistent effort of the will accustoms himself to short and disturbed rest, the signs of distress which the unrefreshed body first feels are modified, and extremely short hours of sleep may become the rule of life. . . .

"In time, sleeplessness acquired by habit becomes a practice which, when the body has arrived at full maturity and more rest from sleep is absolutely demanded, is not easily thrown aside. At such stage the bad habit tells on the life, and *the physician finds no class of patients so difficult to treat successfully, even for mere functional derangements, as the habitually sleepless.* There is about the patient a restless anxiety, an irritability, and a nervous feebleness which no artificial aid can, entirely, subdue. . . .

"In adolescents, even if they be, naturally, of sound constitution and firm build, deficient sleep is a persistent source of mental and bodily exhaustion. It induces pallor, muscular debility, restlessness, and irritability. It interferes with that natural growth and nutrition of the body to which sound sleep so beneficently ministers, and it makes the work and the pleasure of the wakeful day unduly heavy and laborious.

"These remarks apply to members of both the sexes, but they especially apply to girls. The anæmia, bloodlessness, weakness, and hysterical excitability that characterize the young lady of modern life, who is neither well nor ill, are due, mainly, to her bad habit of taking too limited a supply of sleep at irregular hours.

"The feebleness which falls to the lot of the robust who deprive themselves in youth, or who are deprived, of the due amount of sleep, taken in due season, is greatly increased, and is of much more serious moment, when it falls to those who by hereditary taint are disposed to an acute wasting disease—to pulmonary consumption, to name the most familiar example. . . .

"From adolescence on towards the close of that period of age where the body reaches the period when the maturity is attained and the downward course of life is not yet on hand, the strong man can resist sleep often for long periods. He is apt, in consequence, to trespass on the liberty he ventures to take with nature; and when from any cause he chooses to take the liberty, he congratulates himself, perchance, on the impunity with which he is able to violate the natural law. The delusion is not of very long duration. As the middle of the second stage of his career approaches the demand for more sleep becomes more urgent, and happy is he who at this crisis can recall to his service the friend he has deserted.

"If in middle age the habit of taking deficient and irregular sleep be still maintained, every source of depression, every latent form of disease, is quickened and intensified. The sleepless exhaustion allies itself with all other processes of exhaustion, or it kills imperceptibly by a rapid introduction of premature old age, which leads directly to premature dissolution. . . .

"The effect of irregular hours and of deficiency of sleep is developed sometimes in another way.

"When the exhaustion from prolonged sleeplessness is felt it is demonstrated through the heart. Intermittent action of the heart is established, and all the evils belonging to that broken movement are set in train. This state of things is most readily induced in those persons who, while losing their natural rest, are engaged in working against time. Newspaper reporters and night pressmen are very quickly influenced in this manner, and become disabled before they are fully alive to their disablement. They feel at times a strange sensation of faintness or coldness coming over them, as if they were suddenly enveloped in a haziness or obscurity; but, by applying more desperately to their work, they dash the sensation aside until it returns too often to be disposed of so readily. Then they are discovered to be suffering from exhausted brain and irregular circulation.

"Another effect is sometimes witnessed, and is the most distressing of all. It is that the sleeplessness acquired by habit begets sleeplessness. The most extreme insomnia is herewith induced, and the mind, knowing no rest by night or by day, is quickly off its balance. The very idea that sleep will not come under any circumstances, unless it be enticed by powerful narcotics, is itself preventive of all natural repose, and as the dread of the sleeplessness increases other morbid trains of thought arise in rapid succession. Some hypochondriacal monomania seizes the sufferer; he imagines the most improbable accidents are about to happen to him; he is constantly restless; he bites his nails to the quick, or keeps up some peculiar motion of his limbs, a rat-tat on the table or a gesticulatory action of an exaggerated character. A man circumstanced in this manner passes, usually, with steady advance, into insanity—too often into suicide. . . .

"I have said that those who sleep differently and irregularly are more easily affected by direct causes of disease and are less amenable to means of cure. To this should be added the equally important fact that those who are habituated to full and regular sleep are those who recover most readily from sickness. The observation of this truth led Menander to teach that *sleep is the natural cure of all diseases.* It is so. *Sleep reduces fever, quickens nutrition, increases elimination, soothes pain,* and *encourages the healing of wounded surfaces.* Whoever is first to discover the still secret cause of natural sleep *and the mode in which it may be commanded by art, for the service of mankind, will be the greatest healer who has, up to this age, helped to make medicine immortal.*"

The length of time a man can preserve his mental faculties without sleep varies more or less with the constitution, but the inevitable result is delirium before many days. The Chinese punish a certain class of flagrant crimes by constantly teasing the criminal to prevent his sleeping, and it is among the punishments regarded by them with most horror. Historians report that Perseus, the last king of ancient Macedonia, while a prisoner of the Romans, was "done to death" in this way by his guards. They would not permit him to sleep.

When the first Napoleon attempted the conquest of Hayti, Toussaint L'Ouverture, who had become commander-in-chief of the Haytians, could not venture a pitched battle with the battalions of Napoleonic veterans, but had recourse to a less risky though more effective method of warfare. As soon as the French troops got to sleep at night, Toussaint made a feint of attacking them, thus getting them all up and under arms. This was repeated so frequently as effectually to prevent their getting any rest, and in a few weeks an army of thirty thousand veterans, without a single engagement in the field, was reduced to about five thousand effectives, through disease induced mainly, if not entirely, by want of sleep. It is reported that the policy of the Haytian patriot was prosecuted by the insurgents in Cuba in their late war of independence.

Is it not obvious that something goes on during sleep which is a preventative of mania; some change is wrought that could not be wrought until the patient was liberated from the bondage of his worldly environment, and made accessible to influences of some kind which could not approach him while under such bondage, and that those influences are soothing, civilizing, harmonizing, fraternizing, elevating.

The predatory animals, as a rule, seek their prey at night and their repose by day. They differ in this respect from all tamed or domesticated animals. It is also to be observed that they subsist chiefly upon the food of other animals, and are, therefore, ever at war with the whole animal kingdom, not always sparing their own progeny. Like the dangerous classes of human society, they take advantage of the darkness to better conceal their purposes, and for the greater chance of finding their prey asleep or off its guard.

To domesticate or tame a wild animal, it is necessary to win its confidence by protecting it from its predatory fellows and accustoming it to sleep without fear. On the other hand, the domesticated animal soon becomes wild and dangerous if its sleep is disturbed; cows fall off in their yield of milk; hens will not lay; sheep will not fatten.

Wild beasts are always lean, or, rather, never fat, partly, no doubt, if not entirely, because of their precarious livelihood, which compels them to be constantly on the alert by night as well as by day.

The savage tribes, who for the most part lead predatory lives, are so much exposed to surprises that they rarely get regular or sufficient sleep, and take their rest as they take their food, when they can get it, but without periodicity or regularity. This goes far to explain not only why they are savage, but why their average longevity is much less than that of civilized peoples. As they emerge from the savage state they begin to organize into societies for mutual protection, to share one another's burdens, and to secure social privileges, of which regular and abundant sleep is one to which all the others are secondary. That is the "pillar of fire by night" which guides them from a life of barbaric selfishness towards a higher life of mutual forbearance and fraternity. The policeman's rattle is the official symbol of civilization, for upon the forces it rallies to the defence of order we depend for our undisturbed repose during the hours when darkness offers a partial immunity to crime.

The venomous snake, which is the symbol of all which is most detested and detestable in the animal kingdom, never closes its eyes. They are covered with a sort of scale, transparent, like glass, which allows perfect vision, and yet is strong enough to protect the eyes from the ordinary accidents of snake life. While warm-blooded animals shut their eyelids to exclude the light when they sleep and the pupils relax or open, in the serpent this action is reversed—the pupil contracts like a cat's in the sunlight. It is a curiously suggestive and, I believe, a well-authenticated fact, that the most deadly serpents, the *Viperidae* and *Boidae*, are cat-eyed and night-prowlers. Except when thirsty, they will rarely be seen moving about in the daytime. The *Colubridae*, or common, harmless snakes, on the other hand, have round pupils, sleep at night, and are active chiefly during sunlight hours.

Professor W. E. Leonard, of Minneapolis, has given a most interesting account of the pathogenetic effects of what is known in medical literature as *lachesis*. The late Dr. Herring, of Philadelphia, and his brave wife are its hero and heroine. Lachesis is the common name of a deadly poisonous serpent named by Linnæus *Trigonocephalus lachesis,* partly from its lance-shaped head, and partly from one of the Greek Fates, and because of the swift and fatal effects of its bite.

Herring, in his *Condensed Materia Medica,* enumerates *persistent sleeplessness* among the pathogenetic symptoms for which lachesis is a specific, on the homœopathic principle that the hair of the dog that bites will cure, or *similia similibus curantur.* Also, "*children toss about, moaning during sleep.*"

I refer to the venom of the lachesis as a remedial agent, because it is, I believe, a rare, if not the only instance of any deadly serpent's venom having been tested, and its effects upon the human system carefully noted in minute detail, and classified by a professional man eminently qualified for such a task. It will be observed that the most conspicuous effect of this poison is hostility to sleep, and when sleep does intervene it aggravates all other symptoms, as if it and sleep were the deadliest and wholly unreconcilable enemies. It achieves its victories over its victims more swiftly than mere privation of sleep induced by most other causes is supposed to, but in both cases privation of sleep seems to be the one symptom without the concurrence of which none of the others would necessarily be fatal.

When we reflect that the serpent in all ages

has been the symbol of what was most fatal to man's peace; that it was the serpent that first brought temptation and disobedience into the world; that with the Greeks the head of Medusa, with its snaky hair, was the symbol of the paralyzing influence of vice; that Mercury's wand was composed of the figures of two fighting serpents, and that he himself commenced his career as a divinity by stealing the oxen of Apollo; when we reflect that serpent-worship prevails almost universally among savages, who fear the power and cunning of serpents, and try to propitiate them by paying them divine honors; and moreover, if it be true, as there is ample warrant for presuming, "a reason more perfect than reason, and influenced by its partialities, is at work in us when we sleep"; if, as the pagan philosopher affirmed, "the night-time of the body is the day-time of the soul"; if our Father which is in heaven "giveth his beloved in their sleep," how naturally and instinctively we associate the serpent's deadly bite, so fatal to sleep and life, with the fearful curse denounced against the first of the reptiles of whom we have any record, through whose subtlety, temptation and sin first came into the world. Hence perhaps it is that the serpent in the Bible symbolizes every form of temptation to evil or sin, and hence, only in our sleep are the weapons forged with which we can successfully contend with them.

Shakespeare, who was no less unapproachable

for his philosophic insight than as a poet, makes Cæsar say:

"Let me have men about me that are fat;
Sleek-headed men, and *such as sleep o' nights;*
Yond' Cassius has a lean and hungry look;
. . . but I fear him not;
Yet if my name were liable to fear,
I do not know the man I should avoid
So soon as that spare Cassius.
. . . .
Seldom he smiles, and smiles in such a sort,
As if he mock'd himself, and scorn'd his spirit,
That could be mov'd to smile at anything.
Such men as he be never at heart's ease
Whiles they behold a greater than themselves;
And therefore are they very dangerous."

Brutus was selected by the partisans hostile to Cæsar to be the leader in the conspiracy against him, because, as Cassius expressed it:

"He sits high in all the people's hearts:
And that which would appear offence in us,
His countenance, like richest alchemy,
Will change to virtue and to worthiness."

After calling his servant Lucius several times without receiving any reply—it is after midnight and the man is asleep—Brutus exclaims:

"I would it were my fault to sleep so soundly."

In the same scene Lucius is again caught napping. Brutus calls:

"Boy! Lucius!—Fast asleep? It is no matter;
Enjoy the heavy honey-dew of slumber:
Thou hast no figures nor no fantasies,
Which busy care draws in the brains of men;
Therefore thou sleep'st so sound."

When Lucius is gone and leaves Brutus alone, he says:

"Since Cassius first did whet me against Cæsar,
I have not slept.
Between the acting of a dreadful thing
And the first motion, all the interim is
Like a phantasma or a hideous dream:
The Genius and the mortal instruments
Are then in council; and the state of man,
Like to a little kingdom, suffers then
The nature of an insurrection."

The pertinacity with which Shakespeare dwells upon the sleeplessness of Brutus from the time he began to entertain the suspicion that the liberties of Rome depended upon the immediate death of Cæsar, is one of the marvels of this marvellous play. A little later in the piece, when Cassius apologizes for entering and disturbing Brutus's rest, Brutus replies that he has been awake all night. In the same scene Portia, his wife, enters to remonstrate with him:

Brutus. Portia, what mean you . . . now?
It is not for your health thus to commit
Your weak condition to the raw-cold morning.

Portia. Nor for yours neither. You've ungently,
Brutus,
Stole from my bed: and yesternight, at supper,
You suddenly arose, and walk'd about,
Musing and sighing, with your arms across;
And when I ask'd you what the matter was,
You star'd upon me with ungentle looks: .
But with an angry wafture of your hand,
Gave sign for me to leave you: so I did;
Fearing to strengthen that impatience
Which seem'd too much enkindled. . . . Dear my lord,
Make me acquainted with your cause of grief.
Brutus. I am not well in health, and that is all.
Portia. Brutus is wise, and, were he not in health,
He would embrace the means to come by it.
Brutus. Why, so I do.—Good Portia, go to bed.
Portia. Is Brutus sick? . . .
And will he steal out of his wholesome bed, . . .
And tempt the rheumy and unpurgèd air
To add unto his sickness? No, my Brutus;
You have some sick offence within your mind,
Which, by the right and virtue of my place,
I ought to know of: and, upon my knees,
I charm you, by my once-commended beauty,
By all your vows of love, and that one great vow
Which did incorporate and make us one,
That you unfold to me, yourself, your half,
Why you are heavy; and what men to-night
Have had resort to you,—for here have been
Some six or seven, who did hide their faces
Even from darkness.

I am still far from having exhausted all that Shakespeare has to teach us on the subject of sleep or its privation. Whatever takes a deep hold upon a mind like Shakespeare's can always be studied with profit, and the prominence he gave to both in his plays warrants the belief that few of the phenomena of sleep or of sleeplessness escaped his incomparable powers of observation. No one familiar with his plays will often think of sleep as a condition of existence without being reminded of that thrilling soliloquy of Henry IV.:

"How many thousand of my poorest subjects
Are at this hour asleep!—O Sleep, O gentle Sleep,
Nature's soft nurse, how have I frighted thee,
That thou no more wilt weigh my eyelids down,
Nor steep my senses in forgetfulness?
Why rather, Sleep, liest thou in smoky cribs,
Upon uneasy pallets stretching thee,
And hush'd with buzzing night-flies to thy slumber,
Than in the perfum'd chambers of the great,
Under the canopies of costly state,
And lull'd with sounds of sweetest melody?
O thou dull god, why liest thou with the vile
In loathsome beds, and leav'st the kingly couch
A watch case or a common 'larum bell?
Wilt thou upon the high and giddy mast
Seal up the ship-boy's eyes, and rock his brains
In cradle of the rude imperious surge,
And in the visitation of the winds,
Who take the ruffian billows by the top,
Curling their monstrous heads, and hanging them
With deafening clamor in the slippery shrouds,
That, with the hurly, death itself awakes?—

Canst thou, O partial Sleep, give thy repose
To the wet sea-boy in an hour so rude;
And in the calmest and most stillest night,
With all appliances and means to boot,
Deny it to a king? Then, happy low, lie down!
Uneasy lies the head that wears a crown."

Queen Margaret thus brings her curse of the villanous Gloster to a climax:

"No sleep close up that deadly eye of thine,
Unless it be while some tormenting dream
Affrights thee with a hell of ugly devils!"

Lady Percy says to Hotspur:

"Why hast thou lost the fresh blood in thy cheeks
And given my treasures and my rights of thee
To thick-eyed musing and curs'd melancholy

. . . .

Tell me, sweet lord, what is't that takes from thee
Thy stomach, pleasure, and thy *golden sleep?*"

The Abbess in "The Comedy of Errors" says to Adriana:

"The venom-clamors of a jealous woman
Poison more deadly than a mad-dog's tooth.
It seems his sleeps were hinder'd by thy railing:

. . . .

In food, in sport, in life-preserving rest
To be disturb'd, would mad or man or beast."

With exquisite art Shakspeare makes Macbeth expatiate upon the blessedness of "innocent sleep" after his murder of Duncan, and after he had forfeited forever the capacity of enjoying it himself:

> "Methought I heard a voice cry 'Sleep no more!
> Macbeth does murder sleep'—the innocent sleep,
> Sleep that knits up the ravell'd sleave of care,
> The death of each day's life, sore labor's bath,
> Balm of hurt minds, great nature's second course,
> Chief nourisher in life's feast."

Later on in the same play we read:

> "With Him above
> To ratify the work—we may again
> Give to our tables meat, sleep to our nights."

In the first scene of the second act of "The Tempest," when Alonzo notes that several of his companions who escaped from the wreck had suddenly gone to sleep, he says:

> What, all so soon asleep! I wish mine eyes
> Would, with themselves, shut up my thoughts: I find
> They are inclined to do so.
> *Seb.*— Please you, sir,
> Do not omit the heavy offer of it:
> It seldom visits sorrow; when it doth,
> It is a comforter.

Iago, after poisoning the jealous nature of Othello, says:

> "Not poppy, nor mandragora,
> Nor all the drowsy syrups of the world,
> Shall ever medicine thee to that *sweet sleep*
> Which thou ow'dst yesterday."

The Witch, in enumerating the calamities in store for the Sailor in "Macbeth," says:

> "Sleep shall neither night nor day
> Hang upon his pent-house lid;
> He shall live a man forbid."

To fall asleep in a house of worship I fancy to be much less of a reproach than is commonly supposed. To the devout worshipper the tendency of everything in the house of God is, or should be, as in sleep—to separate him from the world. In the degree in which our devotions are unmixed, undiluted with selfish, worldly, and personal considerations, our will is also quiescent as in sleep. "Rousing sermons," stirring pulpit oratory, may stimulate the intellect and keep even the devoutest people wakeful, but it does not follow that they make the exercises of the Sabbath more profitable, at least, to all. The most wide-awake people in church may be in a closer relation with the world than with their Creator, who, in the language of the prophet, may be "near in their mouth and far from their reins."

It is not uncommon for those who have no habit or inclination to sleep during the morning hours of secular days, to be overcome with somnolency in church soon after the devotional exercises are begun, and who find it impossible to derive any edification from them until they have lost themselves for a moment or two in absolute unconsciousness. Then they have no difficulty, sometimes a lively pleasure, in attending to the exercises which follow. The worshipper is then withdrawn from the familiar excitement of customary avocations. It is idle to suppose that in these few moments of repose, upright in his pew, he has rested enough, in the common acceptation of that word, to repair any waste of tissue that would explain the new sense of refreshment that ensues. He has received, in that brief retirement from the world, some reinforcements which manifestly are not dependent upon time or space for their efficacy—spiritual reinforcements, and spiritual reinforcements only. He has removed himself, or been removed, further away, out of sight or hearing or thinking, so to speak, of his phenomenal life, and nearer to the Source of all life.

It was quite a common impression among the ancients that sleepers in temples of religion were more apt to receive divine communications there than elsewhere. Strabo is perhaps our most important pagan authority on this subject. He says:

"In fact, Moses, an Egyptian priest, who possessed a part of the country called (Delta?), left there to go into Judea, having taken a disgust for the institutions of his country. With him parted a great number of men who honored the divinity.. He said and taught that the Egyptians and the Libyans were fools to pretend to represent the divinity in the figures of ferocious or domestic animals; that the Greeks were no wiser when they gave Him the human figure. According to him, divinity was nothing else than that which envelops us—the earth and the sea—to wit, what we call heaven, the world, or nature. Now what sensible man would dare to represent this divinity by an image made on the model of one of us? He required them, therefore, to renounce all manufacture of idols, to limit their honors to divinity by dedicating to it a place and a sanctuary worthy of it without any image. It was necessary also that those who were subjects for happy dreams should come to this sanctuary to sleep, in order to acquire their inspirations for them and for others, for the wise and the just had always to expect from the divinity goods, favors, signs; but this expectation is interdicted to other mortals.

"By this discourse Moses persuaded a large number of men of sense, and led them into the country where is rising to-day the city of Jerusalem."

Pomponius Mela is another pagan writer who speaks of the practice in Italia-Græca of sleeping in temples for the purpose of securing revelations by dreams.

We have already quoted the statement of Iamblichus, "that numbers of sick, by sleeping in the temple of Æsculapius, have had their cure revealed to them in dreams vouchsafed by the god."

Samuel, while a child, slept in the temple of the Lord where the ark of God was. It was there that the Lord called him by name and prepared him to become one of his prophets.*

* 1 Samuel iii. 19.

Among the Hebrews the practice seems to have been quite common. We are told in Luke xi. 36, that Anna the Prophetess, who had been a widow fourscore-and-four years, "departed not from the temple; worshipping with fastings and supplications night and day."

Solomon went to Gibeon to sacrifice; "the people sacrificed only in high places, because there was no house built for the name of the Lord until those days." Gibeon was the great high place, which meant the place where there was a house built for the name of the Lord. It was while there, we are told, that the Lord appeared to Solomon in a dream by night; and because he asked the Lord to give him an understanding heart to judge his people that he might discern between good and evil, and did not ask for riches and long life, the Lord gave him not only for what he asked, but riches and honor as well, "so that there should be no kings like him in all his days," and a contingent promise to lengthen his days.

So in Hosea it is said:

"The Lord hath also a controversy with Judah, and will punish Jacob according to his ways; according to his doings will he recompense him. In the womb he took his brother by the heel; and in his manhood he had power with God: yea, he had power over the angel, and prevailed: he wept, and made supplication unto him: *he found him at Beth-el, and there he spake with us; even the Lord, the God of hosts.*"

It does not seem to have occurred to any of these authorities that this greater accessibility to spiritual influence might have been due only to the more complete abstraction from the world which such a retreat encourages.

Dean Swift, in a letter to Pope, August 30, 1716, says: "I know it was anciently the custom to sleep in temples for those who would consult the oracles. 'Who dictates to me slumbering,'" etc.*

I am indebted to Dr. Carl Abel, a learned German philologist, for a clipping from the Berlin *Woche*, one of the most prominent of German illustrated weeklies, which he accompanies with the following remarks:

"It [the clipping] actually alleges the continuance to this day in a Roman Catholic village near Vienna of the ancient Jewish practice of sleeping in hallowed precincts with a view to being favored with inspired dreams. At Jerusalem it was the temple that promised inspiration; at Vienna, or, rather, at Salmannsdorf, it is a sacred wood. In the ancient dispensation the communication expected was to enable the recipient to discern the tendency of the divine will in a matter of serious import. At present the oracle sought after seems generally to refer to the choice of lottery tickets."

The following is a translation of the clipping from the *Woche*, August 2, 1902:

"HOLY FOREST.—A quite unusual picture may be seen within five minutes' distance of the great city of

* Milton.

Vienna, in the forest of Salmannsdorf. The trees at the entrance of the forest are hung with oil paintings and engravings, etchings, bronzes, marbles, etc.—a real art-gallery created by religious people, among which connoisseurs will recognize many valuable pieces, suffering from exposure to the weather. This place, about which there are many stories current, is considered holy and is called 'Forest Prayer.' Crowds of the superstitious sleep there in the hope of dreaming the lucky numbers to be played for in the Austrian lotteries."

To this it is pleasant to add some wise observations of a Russian lady who has recently published a work of substantial value on the pathology of sleep:

"All the complicated conditions of social existence to which during waking life we are all obliged to conform or to resist, are eliminated during sleep and the psychic life of dreams unrolls freely without the impeding fetters of social laws. It cannot be denied that these social laws, which surround every human existence, sometimes become a heavy burden, and that they develop at the same time a certain hypocrisy in feeling and thought and action, and thus give rise to endless falsehood and deceit. In sleep all this changes. We are delivered from the heavy burden imposed by those vital conditions which by virtue of historical development have gained a certain empire in a given nation or society, but which are very often at the same time not merely opposed to the desires and impulses of men, but even injurious to the development and well-being of individuals who live in the midst of the nation or society. From all these conventional chains we are liberated during sleep and brought, as it were, face to face with nature. During sleep—as the philosophic physiologist, Burdach, remarked—all social differences disappear; and men attain that perfect equality which in the waking state they can only dream of."*

Lord Byron told George Ticknor that he wrote the *English Bards and Scotch Reviewers* at his paternal estate in the country the winter before he set forth on his travels, while a heavy fall of snow was on the ground, and he kept house for a month, during which time he never saw the light of day, rising in the evening after dark and going to bed in the morning before dawn.

What better, what other explanation could be given of the tone, spirit, and purpose of this brutal satire than this systematic and persistent violation of the laws of nature for a whole month, during which time noxious stimulants were to a large extent a substitute for wholesome sleep?

The medical profession throughout the world has generally accepted Hufeland's division of a day of time as incontestably the most rational—that is: eight hours for work, eight hours for sleep, eight hours for nourishment, corporal exercise, and recreation.

Humboldt, of delicate health in his youth, like Napoleon and Leibnitz, is reported to have allowed himself but three hours' sleep in every twenty-

* *Sleep: Its Physiology, Pathology, Hygiene, and Psychology.* By Marie Manaceine, p. 112.

four, and that, despite the enormous activity of his mind, he attained a very advanced age. Lest one should attach undue importance to such an eminent example, I will quote one or two extracts which deserve, I think, to be carefully weighed in the balance against Humboldt's practice, if that practice is correctly reported.

Schmettau, in his Life of Frederick William the Fourth, says, in speaking of Humboldt's *Cosmos*,

> "in which, without any thought of the Creator, he faithfully describes nature and everything which man has been able to prize there, regardless of the Bible, which only exalts the acts of the Creator without occupying itself with the achievements of men. The man who, in combining the results of an existence of eighteen lustres has only succeeded in blaséing himself with his own self-sufficiency and in proudly leaving God on one side, living without thought of Him, cannot yet have penetrated to the sources of wisdom the fruit of which is peace to the soul. The influence which Humboldt has exerted on his age will probably profit no one except the powers which wish to destroy that peace."

G. Menzel, in his *History of Modern Times*, speaking of the *Cosmos*, says:

> "It was in express conflict with the Bible as the Book of Books. In his exposé of the totality of nature there is no veneration nor mention of the Creator. Nature appears there as an indifferent substance which only acquires importance as it is recognized and employed

by man. Humboldt takes no account of the Creator and the essence of things, only of the man who discovers, explains, and invents. He only exalts the human intellect as an explorer, and works entirely in the sense of the Hegelian philosophy, in which God exists only so far as he is the object of the thought of man. Under Humboldt's influence the natural sciences in Germany, with scarcely an exception, were turned against Christianity."

Would Humboldt have left such a deplorable record among his most enlightened contemporaries had he divided his day as recommended by Hufeland?

CHAPTER VII

What is meant by God's resting on the seventh day of creation and enjoining the observance of the Sabbath as a day of rest for his people.

THE faithful student of the Bible may ask, How can one reconcile this theory of sleep with the second of the commandments delivered to Moses, in which we are told that on the expiration of the six days in which God created the heavens and the earth, He *rested the seventh day?* If God *rested,* why should not man rest?

This question might be best answered, perhaps, by another. How can a being of infinite power be conceived of experiencing fatigue, or needing rest in the sense implied in this question? Such a notion of God is not only inconsistent with the necessary and indisputable attributes of the Supreme Being—the *Causa causans;* but, worse than that, it imports either polytheism or atheism.

It was one of the reproaches which the pagans made against the early Christians that they passed every seventh day in effeminate idleness, in imitation of *their wearied God*—a reproach which is not without point, if the God they worshipped was subject to fatigue.

Claudius Rutilius Namatianus, author of an elegiac poem in two books, describing his trip from Rome to Gaul, 416 A.D., speaks of a charming country place he visited on leaving Falerie, the manager in charge of which was a querulous Jew:

"Namque loci querulus curam
Judæus agebat,"—

who scolds him for disturbing the shrubbery and wasting the water.

"We rebuked him" [he says] "as his ignoble race deserved—a shameless people whose practice of circumcision is the root of all absurdities of this ignoble race, who celebrate with all their soul their stupid Sabbath, but with a soul more stupid than their religion, and pass in shameful idleness every seventh day in effeminate *imitation of their wearied God.*"*

Another answer to the question may be found in the second and third verses of the second chapter of Genesis, where we are told that "God finished his work which he had made; and he *rested* on the seventh day from all his work which he had made. And God blessed the seventh day and

*"Reddimus obscenæ convicia debita genti
Quæ genitale caput propudiosa metit,
Radix stultitiæ, cui frigida sabbata cordi,
Sed cor frigidius religione sua:
Septima quæque dies turpi damnata veterno,
Tanquam lassati mollis imago dei."

hallowed it, *because* that *in it he rested* from all his work which God had created and made."

Rest in its ordinary acceptance implies exhaustion of force; a feebleness which if not reinforced must result in death—a condition not thinkable of our Creator. In the case under consideration it could mean nothing of that kind because another and very different reason was distinctly assigned; it was because God had distinguished that from other days of creation by blessing and sanctifying it.

In blessing and sanctifying rest, God certainly did not bless and sanctify idleness, an interruption of growth, a suspension of all productive activities, a temporary death. These are not qualities that merit or invite sanctification, any more than omnipotence is susceptible of fatigue. It is clear that this discrimination of the Sabbath from other days was not to secure physical repose and recuperation, the antithesis and commonly received antidote to fatigue. It was, as we are assured by the divine record, because the people of Israel had been slaves in Egypt—that is, in bondage to sinful habits, propensities, and passions, an inordinate and debasing selfhood from which the Lord had emancipated them. The Sabbath was to be kept to remind them of their great deliverance and of the duties and obligations which that deliverance imposed. It was a new provision for the new spiritual condition to which they had been advanced.

If mere physical repose and functional recuperation is not meant—and such it certainly could not have been—we must look elsewhere for the true significance of a practice or ceremonial of which our Father in heaven set the first example and which He requires all his children to follow.

Happily, Paul the Apostle has thrown some light upon this question, though it was not precisely the subject of which he was treating at the time. In his Epistle to the Hebrews, third and fourth chapters, he says:

While it is said, To-day if ye will hear his voice, harden not your hearts, as in the provocation.

For some, when they had heard, did provoke: howbeit not all that came out of Egypt by Moses.

But with whom was he grieved forty years? was it not with them that had sinned, whose carcasses fell in the wilderness?

And to whom sware he that they should *not enter into his rest,* but to them that believed not?

So we see that *they could not enter in because of unbelief.*

Let us therefore fear, lest, a promise being left us of *entering into his rest,* any of you should seem to come short of it.

For unto us was the gospel preached, as well as unto them: but the word preached did not profit them, not being mixed with faith in them that heard it.

For we which have believed do *enter into rest,* as he said, As I have sworn in my wrath, if they shall enter into my rest: although the works were finished from the foundation of the world.

For he spake in a certain place of the seventh day on this wise, And God did rest the seventh day from all his works.

And in this place again, If they shall enter into my rest.

Seeing therefore it remaineth that some must enter therein, and they to whom it was first preached entered not in because of unbelief:

Again, he limiteth a certain day, saying in David, To-day, after so long a time; as it is said, To-day if ye will hear his voice, harden not your hearts.

For if Jesus had given them rest, then would he not afterward have spoken of another day.

There remaineth therefore a rest to the people of God.

For he that is entered into his rest, he also hath *ceased from his own works*, as God did from his.

Let us labor therefore to enter into that rest, lest any man fall after the same example of unbelief.*

Here it is distinctly stated that the generation which Moses led out of bondage in Egypt was not permitted to enter into God's rest—First, because they do always err in their hearts; secondly, because they have not known God's ways; thirdly, because they had sinned; fourthly, because of unbelief.

Then Paul adds that he and his followers which have believed do enter into rest, and that there remaineth a rest to the people of God "for he that is entered into his rest, he also hath ceased from his own works as God did from his."

* Paul to the Hebrews iii. 14.

When Paul here speaks of himself and his followers entering into rest he says that "they ceased from their own works," not as a ploughman does at shut of day, but "as God did from his." Paul was never more active, never more zealous in the calling wherewith he was called, than at that period of his life when he was inditing these lines in commendation of the rest into which he and his followers had entered.

When we regard—as enlightened theologians usually do—the bondage of the Israelites in Egypt, referred to in Paul's exposition, as a bondage to sin, and their deliverance from it as the beginning of the process of regeneration, we then begin to comprehend the necessity for the prosecution of the work of regeneration represented by the forty years' struggle with trials and temptations in the wilderness, and for a periodical withdrawal from worldly cares and from exposure to worldly temptations, and for the consecration of a portion of our time and thoughts to the entire exclusion of those distractions.

The Lord, in excusing Himself for what He had done to and for the children of Israel in leading them out of Egypt and giving them his statutes and judgments, "which if a man do he shall live by them," added:

> "Moreover, also, I gave them my Sabbath to be a sign between me and them that they might know that I am the Lord that sanctify them."

Sanctification, not idleness, was the great and the exclusive purpose of the Sabbath and its rest. Is not sanctification the purpose of all rest, and is not all rest a detachment from the world, which is only complete in sleep and in death?

Again, in the twenty-eighth verse of the fortieth chapter of the same prophet, he says:

"The everlasting God, the Lord, the Creator of the ends of the earth, *fainteth not, neither is weary*. There is no searching of his understanding. He giveth power to the faint, and to him that hath no might he increaseth strength."

In the fifteenth verse of the thirtieth chapter of Isaiah, the Lord God, the Holy One of Israel, is reported as saying:

"In returning and rest shall ye be saved; in quietness and in confidence shall be your strength: and ye would not."

The most compact definition of the rest which the Sabbath was intended to secure perhaps is given in the fifty-eighth chapter of Isaiah, the spirit of which will be found in the following verses:

"If thou turn away thy foot from doing thy pleasure on my holy day, and call the sabbath a delight, the holy of Jehovah honorable; and shalt honor him, *not doing thine own ways, nor finding thine own pleasure, nor speaking thine own words*: then shalt thou be delightful to Jehovah the Lord, and I will cause thee to ride upon the high places of the earth, and feed thee with the heritage of Jacob."

And here we are confronted by a serious and pregnant inquiry. Is not every incident of our lives which detaches our affections from this world or diminishes the value of all selfish pleasures in our eyes part of that rest which the Sabbath was intended to secure us?

Nothing happens by chance. Nothing is accidental. Neither can we conceive of any waste of divine energy. Everything that occurs we must presume is working the purposes of divine love and wisdom. What, then, is the sanctifying purpose of the innumerable interruptions, disappointments, and defeats of which the earthly lives of the wisest and best, as well as the weakest and basest, experience? What is the compensation we are to expect for our ever-recurring hunger and fatigue, for the pains, the illnesses, disasters in business, involuntary idleness, unwelcome and inconvenient claims upon our time, and unprofitable distractions which we can neither avoid nor enjoy? What else but what our Father in heaven meant when He said of the Israelites to the prophet:

> "Moreover I gave them my sabbaths, to be a sign between me and them, that they might know that I am the Lord; *that I sanctify them.*"*

What are they but sabbaths designed to weaken or break the hold of the world upon us; to impair

* Ezekiel xx. 12.

our natural confidence in our self-sufficiency; to give us his rest from labors that are too engrossing and which prevent our knowing the Lord who is sanctifying it? All trials and tribulations are messengers from heaven sent in love and mercy. All of them, from the least unto the greatest, tend to weaken this world's hold upon us. Do they not all, then, perform, in a degree and more or less frequently, what is manifestly the one great function of sleep?

The Lord has assured us that He is always knocking at every one's door and waiting to be asked to come in and sup with him. What are any of our tribulations but his knocks at our door; his sabbaths that He wishes to sanctify to us? We are prostrated by disease, with alarming uncertainties as to its final result. How rapidly all our worldly interests sink in value as those uncertainties increase; how soon all our worldly ambitions pass from our thoughts like a vision of the night; how readily would we exchange all our wealth or honors for the robust health of the coal-heaver or the hod-carrier. The world's pomps and vanities shrink under trials only less than in sleep, when they entirely disappear for a season; or in death, when they disappear altogether.

May it not be fairly questioned whether the perusal of a fine poem or romance, or the contemplation of a masterpiece of art of any kind, has ever a loftier mission than to release us for a time from this thraldom of our daily cares; to supply us with new and captivating ideals, and make us realize our capacity for the enjoyment of higher modes of existence and nobler pleasures? In other words, are they not handmaidens of sleep? But more on this subject presently.

CHAPTER VIII

Prominence given to the morning hour in the Bible, and its spiritual significance.

I HAVE already referred to the great changes, physical, mental, and moral, which we appear to undergo during the intervals of sleep.

"A man," says Dr. Bushnell, "must be next to a devil who wakes angry. After his unconscious Sabbath he begins another day, and every day is Monday. How beautifully thus we are drawn, by this kind economy of sleep, to the exercise of all good dispositions! The acrid and sour ingredients of evil, the grudges, the wounds of feeling, the hypochondriac suspicions, the black torments of misanthropy, the morose fault-findings, are so far tempered and sweetened by God's gentle discipline of sleep that we do not even conceive how demoniacally bitter they would be if no such kind interruptions broke their spell."

All these experiences are doubtless more or less familiar to everybody; and they give a peculiar significance and importance to many of the most momentous spiritual epochs in the history of our race.

It will be a careless reader of the Bible who will not be struck by the frequency with which epochal events are there reported to have occurred in the morning, and, in many instances, when to all human appearances there could be no reason for naming any time at all for their occurrence, and still less for their occurrence at the time named. The reader will do well to note the extreme importance of the communication in every instance here cited.

We are told that Jacob awoke out of his *sleep* and said: "Surely the Lord is in this place; and I knew it not. And he was afraid, and said, How dreadful is this place. This is none other than *the house of God* and this is the *gate of heaven*."*

> "The Lord said unto Moses, *Rise up early in the morning*, and stand before Pharaoh; lo, he cometh forth to the water; and say unto him, Thus saith the Lord, Let my people go."†

It was *at midnight* that the Lord smote all the first-born in the land of Egypt, but the houses of the children of Israel were passed over. "There shall no plague be upon you to destroy you, when I smite the land of Egypt, *and this day shall be unto you for a memorial and ye shall keep it a feast to the Lord*."‡

On this *fateful night* it was ordered that none

* Genesis xxviii. 16–18. † Exodus viii. 20.
‡ Exodus xii. 14.

of the Israelites were to go out of the door of his house *until the morning.**

The *same night* Pharaoh rose and all his servants and all the Egyptians, and he called up *Moses and Aaron by night,* and said: "Rise up, get you forth from among my people, both ye and the children of Israel: and go serve the Lord as ye have said."† So "it came to pass at the end of four hundred and thirty years, even the self-same day it came to pass that all the hosts of the Lord went out from the land of Egypt. *It is a night of watching unto the Lord* for bringing them out of the land of Egypt: *this same night is a night of watching unto the Lord for all the children of Israel throughout their generations.*"

As nothing in the divine economy is accidental, nor anything in God's word which has not a message for us, we are forced to assume that it was not by accident that the hour of midnight was chosen to smite the first-born of the Egyptians for their obduracy; that the Israelites were forbidden to leave their houses that night; and that Pharaoh called upon Moses and Aaron at night to rise up, take his people, and go and serve the Lord as he wished. Regarded as an ordinary concession from a sovereign to a refractory class of his subjects, the wonder is why this judgment upon the Egyptians and this deliverance of the Israelites should have been wrought in the night,

* Exodus xii. 22. † Exodus xii. 31.

when to the natural eye there appears no reason why it might not have been conducted more conveniently for all parties by daylight.

When Pharaoh and his host pursued the children of Israel and went in after them into the midst of the sea, "it came to pass *in the morning watch* that the Lord looked forth upon the host of the Egyptians through the pillar of fire and of cloud and discomfited the host of the Egyptians. . . . And Moses stretched forth his hand over the sea, and the sea returned in its strength *when the morning appeared*. . . . And the waters returned and covered the chariots and the horsemen, even all the host of Pharaoh that went after them into the sea. There remained not so much as one of them. . . . And Israel saw the great work which the Lord did upon the Egyptians, and the people feared the Lord; and they believed in the Lord and in his servant Moses."

When the children of Israel were being led out of their bondage to the Egyptians "The Lord went before them by day in a pillar of cloud, to lead them the way; and by night in a pillar of fire, to give them light; *to go by day and night.*

"He took not away the pillar of cloud by day, nor the pillar of fire by night, from before the people."*

The night was no more to be wasted than the

* Exodus xiii. 22.

day. But how was it to be improved? Not merely by fleeing from Egyptians, but from their bondage to sins they were leaving behind them.

In what way, then, did they prosecute their journey by night? Of course they could not march day and night. That was physically impossible. Besides, we read continually of their camping in different places. They camped at Elim; they were a long time camped at Rephidim. Then they were camped before Mount Sinai, where they received through Moses the Commandments and a code of laws. There they tarried a long time. After many years they abode in Kadish, where Miriam died and was buried. Later at Mount Hor they mourned thirty days for Aaron, who died and was buried there.

But the Lord went before them all this time. His work with them was not suspended by night any more than by day.

Who can read these citations, thus grouped together, without wondering that the time when the events to which they refer occurred is so uniformly given, when, to all appearance, it is of no earthly importance? The thoughtful reader will be forced to the conclusion that the data in question were either idle and superfluous or that the events referred to had some essential and inevitable relation to the particular time of their occurrence.

The first theory can only be accepted by those who dispute the supernatural origin of the Word.

Those who açcept the other theory and have read these verses, will have no difficulty in divining what, in the eyes of the writer, that essential and inevitable relation is.

When the children of Israel murmured against Moses and Aaron and pined in the wilderness for the flesh-pots of Egypt, the Lord promised Moses to rain bread from heaven for them.

"And Moses and Aaron said unto all the children of Israel, At even, then ye shall know that the Lord hath brought you out from the land of Egypt.

"And *in the morning, then ye shall see the glory of God."**

The Israelites, we are told, subsisted for the next forty years of their wanderings in the wilderness upon this manna sent from heaven. They were instructed to gather it, every man according to his eating, but said Moses, "Let no man leave of it until the morning." This bread sent them from heaven was to be eaten at night; "And in the morning," adds Moses, "ye shall see the glory of God."

The Lord's bread is the bread of life—bread for the soul as well as the body.

No circumstance connected with the proclamation of the Ten Commandments can be treated with indifference or as of secondary importance. Here is the account of that event as recorded in

*Exodus xvi. 6, 7.

the twenty-fourth chapter of Exodus, and the reader will please note the time selected for the most important message perhaps that was ever given to our race:

"The Lord said unto Moses, Hew thee two tables of stone like unto the first: and I will write upon the tables the words that were on the first tables, which thou breakest. And be ready *by the morning*, and *come up in the morning* unto Mount Sinai and present thyself there to me on the top of the Mount. . . . And he hewed two tables of stone like unto the first; and Moses *rose up early in the morning* and went up unto Mount Sinai, as the Lord had commanded him, and took in his hand two tables of stone. And the Lord descended in the cloud, and stood with him there, and proclaimed the name of the Lord."

When the Lord gave Moses the tables of stone and the law and the commandment that he might teach them, "Moses wrote all the words of the Lord, and rose up *early in the morning*, and builded an altar under the mount, and twelve pillars, according to the twelve tribes of Israel. . . . And he took the book of the covenant, and read in the audience of the people: and they said, All that the Lord hath spoken will we do, and be obedient."*

When Hannah, and Elkanah her husband, went to the high-priest Eli, and obtained his blessing upon their petition that she might become a mother, "her countenance was no more sad. And

* Exodus xxiv. 4-7.

they rose up in the morning early, and worshipped before the Lord, and returned to their house to Ramah."*

When the Philistines insisted that David should not go down with them to the battle, Achish told David: "I know that thou art good in my sight, as an angel of God; notwithstanding the princes of the Philistines have said, He shall not go up with us to the battle. Wherefore now rise up *early in the morning* with the servants of thy lord that are come with me: and as soon as ye be *up early in the morning, and have light,* depart. So *David rose up early,* he and his men, to depart *in the morning,* to return into the land of the Philistines.†

We are told that "David's heart smote him after that he had numbered the people. And when David *rose up in the morning,* the word of the Lord came unto the prophet Gad, David's seer, saying, Go and speak unto David, Thus saith the Lord: I offer thee three things; choose thee one of them, that I may do it unto thee."‡

When the Philistines captured the ark of God from the Hebrews, they brought it into the house of Dagon and set it by Dagon. *Early the following morning,* Dagon was fallen upon his face to the ground before the ark of the Lord. The Philistines then sat Dagon again in his place

* 1 Samuel i. 19. † 1 Samuel xxix. 9.
‡ 2 Samuel xxiv. 10.

beside the ark of God, "and when they arose *early on the morrow morning,* behold Dagon was fallen upon his face to the ground before the ark of the Lord, and the head of Dagon and both the palms of his hands lay cut off upon the threshold, only the stump of Dagon was left him."*

In both these instances, the prostration of Dagon, and finally his mutilation, occurred *in the night-time,* and when the Hebrews, to whose advantage the idol's overthrow inured, were presumably asleep.

One of the most important and pathetic colloquies with a sovereign ever reported was that which Samuel the Prophet had with Saul, the King of Israel, because of his disobedience, finally resulting in Saul's downfall and the establishment of the dynasty of David, from which Jesus the Christ was begotten.

Saul had offended the Lord "for having turned back from following and performing his commandments." His offence was reported *in the night* to Samuel, who rose early to meet Saul *in the morning.*

"Saul said to him, Blessed be thou of the Lord: I have performed the commandment of the Lord. And Samuel said, What meaneth then this bleating of the sheep in mine ears, and the lowing of the oxen which I hear? And Saul said, They have brought them from the Amalekites: for the people spared the best of the

* I Samuel v. 5.

sheep and of the oxen, to sacrifice unto the Lord thy God; and the rest we have utterly destroyed.

"Then Samuel said unto Saul, Stay, and I will tell thee *what the Lord hath said to me this night.* And he said unto him, Say on. And Samuel said, Though thou wast little in thine own sight, wast thou not made the head of the tribes of Israel? And the Lord anointed thee king over Israel; and the Lord sent thee on a journey, and said, Go and utterly destroy the sinners the Amalekites, and fight against them until they be consumed. Wherefore then didst thou not obey the voice of the Lord, but didst fly upon the spoil, and didst that which was evil in the sight of the Lord? And Saul said unto Samuel, Yea, I have obeyed the voice of the Lord, and have gone the way which the Lord sent me, and have brought Agag the king of Amalek, and have utterly destroyed the Amalekites. But the people took of the spoil, sheep and oxen, the chief of the devoted things, to sacrifice unto the Lord thy God in Gilgal. And Samuel said, Hath the Lord as great delight in burnt offerings and sacrifices as in obeying the voice of the Lord? Behold, to obey is better than sacrifice, and to hearken than the fat of rams. For rebellion is as the sin of witchcraft, and stubbornness is as idolatry and teraphim. Because thou hast rejected the word of the Lord, he hath also rejected thee from being king. And Saul said unto Samuel, I have sinned: for I have transgressed the commandment of the Lord, and thy words: because I feared the people, and obeyed their voice. Now therefore, I pray thee, pardon my sin, and turn again with me, that I may worship the Lord. And Samuel said unto Saul, I will not return with thee: for thou hast rejected the word of the Lord, and the Lord hath rejected thee from being king over Israel."

The prophet Ezekiel tells us that "it came to pass in the twelfth year of captivity, that one that had escaped out of Jerusalem came unto me saying, The city is smitten. Now the hand of the Lord had been upon me in the evening, before he that was escaped came; and *he had opened my mouth, until he came to me in the morning;* and my mouth was opened, and I was no more dumb." *

This was the beginning of the most impressive message ever delivered by Ezekiel. It was to show how and by what tribulations men who with their mouth show much love but their heart goeth after their gain, are sometimes made to know that the author of such messages was the Lord.

It is important to notice that Ezekiel's mouth was opened, and he was no more dumb in the morning because the hand of the Lord had been upon him in the evening.

"It is of the Lord's mercies," says the prophet, "that we are not consumed, because his compassions fail not. They are *new every morning;* great is thy faithfulness." †

King David sings:

"My voice shalt thou hear *in the morning,* O Lord, *in the morning* will I direct my prayers unto thee and will keep watch." ‡

* Ezekiel xxxiv. 21. † Lamentations iii. 22, 23.
‡ Psalm v.

"My soul fleeth unto the Lord before the *morning watch;* I say, before the *morning watch.*" *

"Thou hast proved and visited my heart in the *night* season; thou hast tried me and shalt find no weakness in me: for I am utterly purposed that my mouth shall not offend." †

"Sing praises unto the Lord, O ye saints of his, and give thanks to his holy name. For his anger is but for a moment; In his favor is life: Weeping may tarry for the night, But joy cometh *in the morning.*" ‡

"As for me, let me behold thy face in righteousness: Let me be satisfied, *when I awake,* with thy likeness." §

John, the child of Elizabeth, was proclaimed by his father Zacharias as "the prophet of the Highest," who was to go "before the face of the Lord to prepare his ways and give knowledge of salvation unto his people," "whereby," he adds, "the Day Spring from on high hath visited us, to shine upon them that sit in darkness and the *shadow* of death; to guide our feet in the way of peace." ‖

So in Job: "Hast thou commanded the morning since thy days began, and caused the *day spring* to know its place; that it might take hold of the ends of the earth, and the wicked be shaken out of it." ¶

Why on both of these most important occasions is such importance given to the dawn or springtime of the day?

* Psalm cxxx. † Psalm xvii. 3. ‡ Psalm xxx. 4, 5.
§ Psalm xvii. 15. ‖ Luke i. 79. ¶ Job xxxviii. 12.

Does it mean anything more to us than any other part of the day would have meant to us?

It was in reference to precisely this event that the Angel Gabriel said to Mary, "No word from God shall be void of power."*

The Lord Jesus was buried in the evening and was raised on the third day in the morning.

It was on the first day of the week that Mary Magdalen came *early while it was yet dark* to the sepulchre and saw the stone had been taken away from the sepulchre. This led to her being the first to see Jesus and to receive the first communication that was made by Him to the human race after his crucifixion.†

It was *early in the morning* that Jesus came into the temple, and all the people came to Him, and He sat down and taught them.‡

To the angel of the church at Pergamum—"To him that overcometh, to him will I give of the hidden manna and I will give him a white stone, and upon the stone a new *name* written which no one knoweth but he that receiveth it. And I will give him the *morning* star." §

By the Morning Star, the Lord himself, of course, is meant.‖

* Luke i. 37. † Mark xvi. 2. ‡ John viii. 2. § Rev. ii. 12.

‖ "I am the root and offspring of David, the bright and Morning Star."—Apoc. xxii. 16.

"The God of Israel said, the Rock of Israel spake to me: one that ruleth over men righteously, that ruleth in the fear of God. He shall be as the *light of the morning* when the sun riseth, a morning without clouds."—2 Samuel xxiii. 3, 4.

Nicodemus, a man of the Pharisees and a ruler of the Jews, came to Jesus *by night* to ask how a man could be born again when he is old.*

Subsequently at the Crucifixion, and when Joseph of Arimathea had obtained permission of Pilate to take away the body of Jesus, "there came also Nicodemus (he who at the first came to him by night), bringing a mixture of myrrh and aloes."

It is significant that the seemingly unimportant fact that the first visit of Nicodemus to Jesus was *by night* should be here recalled, when Nicodemus appears to assist at our Saviour's burial.

When the Lord promised Solomon long life and riches because, instead of asking for them, he had asked for an understanding heart to judge the people and discern between good and evil, which prayer also was gratified, Solomon awoke, and behold it was a dream in *the night*.†

> "I will praise the Lord, who hath given me counsel; yea, my reins instruct me in the *night* seasons." ‡
>
> "Weeping may tarry for the night, but joy cometh in the morning." §

Though upon a mystery of this character the Word is the highest authority that can be appealed

* John iii. 4. † 1 Kings iii. 15.
‡ Psalm xvi. 7. § Psalm xxx. 5.

to, yet, unless confirmed to some extent by the experience and judgment of men making no claim to supernatural inspiration, it might fail to produce conviction even in minds professing the most absolute faith in revelation.

Of such confirmation there is a great abundance, but here it will be necessary to refer only to three or four, but such as will make up in weight for numbers.

Dante speaks of

"... the hour when her sad lay begins,
The little swallow, near unto the morning,
Perchance in memory of her former woes,
And when the mind of man a wanderer is
More from the flesh and less by thought imprisoned
Almost prophetic in its vision is." *

This theory of morning dreams is in accord with, and no doubt an allusion to, what some call a superstition, but which would be more respectfully described as a conviction among the ancients that *somnium post somnum efficax est atque eveniet sive bonum sit sive malum;* a conviction which Ovid perpetuated in the following lines:

"Namque sub Aurora dormitante lucerna
Somnia quo cerni tempore vera solent." †

The truth of morning dreams, as affirmed in the lines above cited from Dante, was the happy in-

* *Purgatorio* ix. ii.

† *Heroides Epist.* xix. 195.

spiration of the following lines of the late T. W. Parsons, written on the death of his wife's cousin:

"PRESSO AL MATTINO DEL VOR SI SOGNA.—*Dante*

"Love, let's be thankful we are past the time
When griefs are comfortless; and, though we mourn,
Feel in our sorrow something now sublime,
And in each tear the sweetness of a kiss.
Weep on and smile then: for we know in this, O
Our immortality, that nothing dies
Within our hearts, but something new is born;
And what is roughly taken from our eyes
Gently comes back *in visions of the morn*
When dreams are truest."

Milton, invoking his heavenly muse, Ourania, says:

"On evil days though fallen and evil tongues,
In darkness and with darkness compassed round,
And solitude; yet not alone while thou
Visit'st my slumbers nightly or when morn
Purples the east."

Pope, in his *Temple of Fame,* founded upon Chaucer's *House of Fame,* says:

"A balmy sleep had charmed my cares to rest,
And love itself was banished from my breast
(*What time the morn mysterious visions brings*
While purer slumbers spread their golden wings);
A train of phantoms in wild order rose,
And joined, this intellectual scene compose."

Dryden, in his version of *The Tale of the Nun's Priest,* says:

> " Believe me, madam, morning dreams foreshow
> Th' event of things, and future weal and woe."

Virgil tells us that when his hero Æneas was laying the foundations of the Roman Empire in Latium and was much disturbed by the anxieties which beset him, having laid down his weary limbs to give them some long-needed rest, Tiber, the river god, appeared to him, encouraged him not to flinch from his purpose, not to be dismayed by threats of hostility, but with the first setting stars to offer prayers to Juno and by suppliant vows vanquish her resentment and threats, assuring him finally of his success. When the river god had finished he hid himself in the deep lake, while Æneas *at the dawn of day awoke and proceeded to put up to him a prayer of thanks,* with promises to rely upon his aid and to sacrifice upon his altars.

It is a very curious fact, and very proper to be noted in this place, that morning prayers and adorations among the early Romans were put up to the celestial gods, and those of the evening to the infernal.

CHAPTER IX

Our external and our internal memory—Coleridge's "body terrestrial" and "body celestial"—The operations of our non-phenomenal life presumably as important as those of our phenomenal life.

WHENEVER we seriously exercise our reasoning faculties we abstract ourselves from the phenomenal world, and just in proportion to the profundity of our thought, or the degree of our interest in the subject of our meditations, will be the completeness of our abstraction. Few realize that the mind while in that state has nothing more to do with the external world than a mill has to do with producing, shelling, or transporting the grain that is thrown into its hopper. The mill only grinds what is put into it. The rapidity of the mind's action is so great that we have no faculties capable of perceiving when the several operations of the mind, memory, and will begin and end in reaching any conclusion. The fingers of the musician seem to run over the keys of the piano with the rapidity of lightning, but the will, mind, and memory act independently at every note. The will indicates the note to be produced, the memory reports the key that produces that note, the mind selects the proper finger and directs that note to be struck. There the mind would rest if the will and the memory did not suggest another note. This process is repeated throughout the score, until the tune is finished. The mind is a servant of the will, of which the memory is a messenger. Through them the mind is occupied with phenomenal life. Suspend the action of the external memory, however, and then the mind works independently of the external or phenomenal world, and that we suppose to be its condition in sleep.

"Near the Temple of the Muses, built by Ardatus, son of Vulcan," Pausanias tells us, "there is an ancient altar which Ardatus is reported to have dedicated. Upon this altar they sacrifice to the Muses and to Sleep, asserting that *Sleep, above all the deities, is friendly to the Muses.*"

Some modern metaphysicians insist that we are endowed with a subjective and objective mind and corresponding memories. The difference between the two memories would be that we should employ the word "memory" when we wish to designate the subjective intelligence, and the word "recollection" to designate the objective intelligence. Memory in this sense is the active retention and distinct recognition of past ideas in the mind, while recollection is the power of recalling—of re-collecting ideas which have once been in the mind but are for the time being forgotten.

Subjective memory is regarded as retaining all ideas, however superficially they may have been impressed on the objective mind, and it admits of no variation of power in individuals.*

This notion of a subjective memory corresponds in the main with what Sir William Hamilton designated as "mental latency," holding that all recollection consisted in rescuing from the storehouse of latent memory some part of its treasure. He assumed latent memory to be perfect, but while he considered it a normal mental process to elevate a part of the latent treasures of the mind above the plane of consciousness, he recognizes the fact that it is only under the most abnormal conditions that the whole content of the magazine of latent intelligence can be brought to light. He says:

> "The second degree of latency exists when the mind contains certain systems of knowledge or certain habits of action which it is wholly unconscious of possessing in its ordinary state, but which are revealed to consciousness in certain extraordinary exaltations of its powers. The evidence on this point shows that the mind frequently contains whole systems of knowledge which, though in our normal state they may have faded into absolute oblivion, may, in certain abnormal states—as madness, febrile delirium, somnambulism, catalepsy, etc.—flash into luminous consciousness, and even throw into the shade of unconsciousness those

* *A Scientific Demonstration of the Future Life*, by Thomas J. Hudson, p. 212.

other systems by which they had for a long period been eclipsed, and even extinguished. For example, there are cases in which the extinct memory of whole languages was suddenly restored, and—what is even still more remarkable—in which the faculty was exhibited of accurately repeating, in known or unknown tongues, passages which were never within the grasp of conscious memory in the normal state. This degree, this phenomenon of latency, is one of the most marvellous in the whole compass of philosophy."

He then cites some most remarkable instances demonstrative of the perfection of subjective memory.

Both of these philosophers were, consciously or unconsciously, indebted, no doubt, for whatever is true—and there is much in both that is true—to Swedenborg. His theory of a dual memory is more profound, more philosophical, and more comprehensive than either. He says:

"It is scarce known to any one at this day, that every man has two memories—one exterior, the other interior; and that the exterior is proper to his body, but the interior proper to his spirit. . . .

"These two memories are altogether distinct from each other; to the exterior memory, which is proper to man during his life in the world, appertain all expressions by language, also all objects of which the senses take cognizance, and likewise the sciences which relate to the world: to the interior memory appertain the ideas of spirit, which are of the interior sight, and all rational things, from the ideas whereof thought itself exists. That these things are distinct from each other is unknown to man, as well because he does not reflect thereupon, as because he is incorporate, and cannot so easily withdraw his mind from corporeal things.

"Hence it is that men, during their life in the body, cannot discourse with each other but by languages distinguished into articulate sounds, and cannot understand each other unless they are acquainted with those languages; the reason is, because this is done from the exterior memory; whereas, spirits * converse with each other by a universal language distinguished into ideas, of their thought, and thus can converse with every spirit, of whatsoever language or nation he may have been; because this is done from the interior memory; every man, immediately after death, comes into the comprehension of this universal language, because he comes into this interior memory, which is adapted to his spirit.

"The speech of words, as just intimated, is the speech proper to man; and indeed, to his corporeal memory; but a speech consisting of ideas of thought is the speech proper to spirits; and, indeed, to the interior memory, which is the memory of spirits. It is not known to men that they possess this interior memory, because the memory of particular or material things, which is corporeal, is accounted every thing, and darkens that which is interior; when, nevertheless, without interior memory, which is proper to the spirit, man would not be able to think at all.

* "Spiritus inter se loquantur per linguam universalem, in ideas, quales sunt ipsius cogitationis, distinctam et sic quod conversari possint cum unoquovis spiritu cujuscumque linguæ et nationis in mundo fuerat."—*Arcana Coelestia*, § 1772.

"Whatsoever things a man hears and sees, and is affected with, these are insinuated, ***as to ideas and final motives or ends,*** into his interior memory, without his being aware of it, and there they remain, so that not a single impression is lost, although the same things are obliterated in the exterior memory; the interior memory, therefore, is such, that there are inscribed in it all the particular things, yea, the most particular, which man has at any time thought, spoken, and done, yea, which have appeared to him only shadowy, with the most minute circumstances, from his earliest infancy to extreme old age: man has with him the memory of all these things when he comes into another life, and is successively brought into all recollection of them; this is the Book of his Life (*Liber ejus Vitae*), which is opened in another life, and according to which he is judged; all final motives or ends of his life, which were to him obscure; all that he had thought, and likewise all that he had spoken and done, as derived from those ends, are recorded, to the most minute circumstances, in that Book, that is, in the interior memory, and are made manifest before the angels, in a light as clear as day, whensoever the Lord sees good to permit it: this has at times been shown me, and evidenced by so much and various experience, that there does not remain the smallest doubt concerning it.*

* Referring to a singular experience which fell under his own observation while a student at Göttingen, S. T. Coleridge makes a comment which warrants us in supposing that he was, consciously or unconsciously, indebted to Swedenborg for it. He says:

"This fact—it would not be difficult to adduce several of a similar kind—contributes to make it even probable that all thoughts are in themselves imperishable; and that if the intelligent faculty should be rendered more compre-

" Men, during their abode in the world, who are principled in love to the Lord, and in charity toward their neighbor, have with themselves, and in themselves, angelic intelligence and wisdom, but hidden in the inmost of their interior memory; which intelligence and wisdom can by no means appear to them, *before they put off things corporeal;* then the memory of particulars spoken of above is laid asleep, and they are awakened to the interior memory, and afterward to the angelic memory itself.*

" A certain spirit, recently deceased, was indignant at not being able to remember more of the things which he had knowledge of during his life in the body, sorrow-

hensive it would require only a differently apportioned organization — the body celestial instead of the body terrestrial — to bring before every human soul the collective experience of its whole past. And this, perchance, is the Book of Judgment, in the dread hieroglyphics of which every idle word is recorded. Yea, in the very nature of a living spirit, it may be more possible that heaven and earth should pass away than that a single act, a single thought, should be loosened or lost from that living chain of causes with all the links of which, conscious or unconscious, the free-will, our only absolute self, is co-extensive and co-present."—*Biographia Literaria,* Coleridge's Works, Harper & Brothers, 1853, vol. iii. p. 229.

*" The French army at this time," says Count La Vallette, who was serving with it in Egypt, under the first Napoleon, " was remarkably free from any feeling of religion." The Count tells a curious anecdote of a French officer who was with him on a boat which was nearly wrecked. The officer said the " Lord's Prayer " from beginning to end. When the danger was over he was much ashamed, and apologized thus: " I am thirty-eight years old, and I have never uttered a prayer since I was six. I cannot understand how it came into my head just then, for I declare that at this moment it would be impossible for me to remember a word of it."

ing on account of the delight which he had lost, and with which he had formerly been particularly gratified; but he was informed, that in reality he had lost nothing, and that he then knew all and every thing which he had ever known, but that in another life it was not allowable for him to call forth such things to observation; and that he should be satisfied to reflect, that it *was now in his power to think and speak much better and more perfectly, without immersing his rational principle, as before, in the gross, obscure, material, and corporeal things which were of no use in the kingdom to which he was now come;* and that *those things which were in the kingdom of the world, were left behind, and he had now whatever conduced to the use of eternal life,* whereby he might be blessed and happy; thus that it was a proof of ignorance to believe, that in another life there is any loss of intelligence in consequence of not using the corporeal memory, *when the real case is, that in proportion as the mind is capable of being withdrawn from things sensual and corporeal, in the same proportion it is elevated into things celestial and spiritual.*" *

Speaking of the punishments o. some of the evil spirits in hell, Swedenborg says:

"Wondering that they were so severely punished, I perceived that it was *because their crime was of so enormous a kind, arising from the necessity there is that man should sleep in safety, since otherwise the human race must necessarily perish.* I was also made aware that the same thing occurs, although man is ignorant of the fact, in reference to others, whom these spirits endeavor by their artifices to assault during sleep; for unless

* *Arcana Coelestia,* vol. i. §§ 2469–2479.

it be given to converse with spirits, being with them by internal sense, it is impossible to hear, and much more to see, such things, notwithstanding they happen alike to all. The Lord is particularly watchful over man during sleep. *Dominus quam maxime custodit hominem cum dormit.*" *

" Some, by a peculiar mercy, are prepared for heaven by deep sleep and by dreams which infest them in sleep." †

" Others have loved the world; but they are kept in a state of sleep until the delight of the world has been lulled." ‡

" When corporal and voluntary things are quiescent the Lord operates." §

" There is no separation of evil but through its quiescence, nor does it quiesce except from the Lord, and when it thus quiesces goods inflow from the Lord." ‖

We find in the passages here cited:

First. A recognition of the existence in man of two mnemonical functions, each quite distinct from the other; one which takes note of all our thoughts and acts having an apparent bearing upon our external or phenomenal life in this world; the other, which not only takes note of those events, but which takes note also of the moral quality, of the ultimate end in which such thoughts or acts originated.

Secondly. That while some of the impressions which are recorded in what Swedenborg

* *Arcana Coelestia*, vol. i. 959. † *Spiritual Diary*, 427.
‡ *Spiritual Diary*, 4199. § *Arcana Coelestia*, 933.
‖ *Arcana Coelestia*, 1581.

calls the external memory are ultimately obliterated, all which are recorded in what he calls the internal memory remain, to the most minute particular and shade, from the earliest infancy, and are absolutely imperishable.

Thirdly. That as in the spiritual world there are no limitations of time, space, or sense, all communication is, not by the language of words, as in the phenomenal world, but by the ideas which phenomena express or represent, and as ideas are not subject to any of the limitations of time, space, or sense, the end or final purpose of our thoughts or acts are all that leave a permanent impression, just as the story or the thought is all that is left on the reader's mind by the printed page. In the words of Swedenborg, "Actions have their quality from the thoughts, as thoughts have their quality from the ends purposed."

Fourthly. That in proportion as man puts off "things corporeal," as he is emancipated from his material, sensual, worldly thrall, he is awakened to a perception of the intelligence and wisdom stirred up in his interior memory.

There is nothing in our sacred writings, nor, I believe, in any man's experience, which can be said to conflict with or render improbable either of these propositions. Be that as it may, from what we may fairly claim to know from our own experience and observation of the phenomena of sleep, and from what we are bound to infer from the teachings of the sacred writings of all sects and nations of most considerable acceptance throughout the world, and especially from the Christian's Bible, it seems impossible to resist the conclusion that the final purposes of our creation and existence, of our *esse* and our *existere*, are not only as operative during our sleeping as during our waking hours, and that a work is being wrought in us, a process is going on in us, during those hours, which is not and cannot be wrought so effectually, if at all, at any other time; that we are spiritually growing, developing, ripening more continuously, while thus shielded from the distracting influences of the phenomenal world, than during the hours in which we are absorbed by them; that, in the language of the pagan philosopher, "the night-time of the body is the daytime of the soul." Our phenomenal life has its specific lessons for us. Why should not our non-phenomenal life also have its specific lessons for us? Why should we doubt that it is in sleep that God "openeth the ears of men and sealeth their instruction, that he may withdraw man from his purpose and hide pride from man," and "that he may keep back his soul from the pit"? Does not all that we know of sleep, and of its effects upon character, tend to confirm every line and every word of this definite and unconditional and authoritative statement of Job's sympathizing friend? If there is a single precept of our faith more frequently urged and insisted upon by the Christian Church than any other it is the necessity of "overcoming the world." The devil is called the prince of this world. He boasted of the fact to Jesus. The "world" is a synonym for all sorts of sensual lusts and pleasures, and for all undue greed for wealth, dignities, and honors. To overcome the world, to rise superior to its temptations, so that they shall not corrupt our life or blind our judgment, is uniformly presented to us by the Christian Church, as it has been by the most enlightened pagan sects, as the supreme end and purpose of our life in the flesh. Is it not precisely the function of sleep to give us for a portion of every day in our lives a respite from worldly influences which, uninterrupted, would deprive us of the instruction, of the spiritual reinforcements necessary to qualify us to turn our waking experience of the world to the best account without being overcome by them? It is in these hours that the plans and ambitions of our external, worldly life cease to interfere with or obstruct the flow of the divine life into the will. And in these hours may we not be, is it not more than probable that we are, in the society of those "ministering spirits" referred to by Paul "who are sent forth to do service for the sake of them that shall inherit salvation"?

The moral distinction between lower animals and man is curiously illustrated in the character of their sleep. A man ordinarily awakens slowly from a deep sleep; he does not for a time realize where he is; he seems to be more or less dazed and not entirely satisfied with the change which seems to him to have taken place. He is apt to act for a few moments as though he had been in a place or society which he was reluctant to leave. As Charles Lamb expressed it, he wishes to lie a little longer to digest his dreams.

A sleeping dog, however, will hear a noise which his master, though by his side, awake, will not hear, and in an instant is in as full possession of all his faculties as if he had not been sleeping. He betrays no evidence of having reluctantly parted with pleasant company or pleasant occupations. And why should he? He has no affections for his kind when awake for which he would sacrifice a bone, though he did not wish it himself.

Is not this precisely what we should expect from the psychical difference of the dog from the man? And does it not warrant the conclusion that when a man is sleeping his condition and associations are as different from a dog's as they are while awake?

CHAPTER X

In sleep we die daily—God alone is life—All causes are spiritual—All phenomena are results—Scipio's dream—Sleep and death twins.

HAVING, as I think, established at least a violent presumption that something of supreme importance is being operated within us during our sleeping hours; that that something concerns our spiritual training and development; and that this view is countenanced, not only by some of the most eminent thinkers of all time, but by what Christians call the Word of God; may we not penetrate a little further into the mysteries of those consecrated hours?

We are warranted in saying that the constituents of every human being are either material or spiritual, either body or soul. No one has any attributes or qualities that do not come under one or the other of these rubrics. Neither can it be successfully disputed that all matter is inert, is incapable of initiating or of arresting motion; that it can neither be increased nor diminished in volume. Its arrangement or form may be changed, but not its quantity. It has, therefore, no life in itself, though, like a house or a garment, it may be the habitation of life of what we call the soul, or spirit.

It is true that the tree drops its fruit and its leaves in their season, but neither tree, leaf, nor fruit dies; they merely pass into a new form of life, as man is presumed to do when his heart ceases to beat. This habitation returns to its elements, or some other form, neither increased nor impaired in quantity by the change. In the language of Juvenal:

> "Mors sola fatetur
> Quantula sint hominum corpuscula."

But what becomes of the tenant? We neither know nor can conceive of anything having occurred to the soul more certain than, or beyond the fact, that it has been emancipated from the restrictions of its prison-house and set free to do, be, or become whatever it has been prepared for becoming during its earthly confinement.

This spirit was all of the man that was or could have been substantial to him. It possessed and represented all he had or knew of life. It was all there was or is of any one's *I am*.

> "There's not the smallest orb which thou behold'st,
> But in his motion like an angel sings,
> Still quiring to the young-ey'd cherubins:
> Such harmony is in immortal souls;
> *But, whilst this muddy vesture of decay*
> *Doth grossly close it in, we cannot hear it.*" *

* "Merchant of Venice," act v. scene I.

Milton describes the death of Jesus as

> "a death like sleep;
> A gentle drifting to immortal life." *

So when Adam communicated to Eve the conditions upon which they were to leave Paradise, the poet adds:

> "For God is also in sleep, and dreams advise."

All life emanates from our Creator, who is life itself, and necessarily the source of all life—a doctrine I was gratified to find dogmatically and most impressively stated quite recently by the head of the most numerous division of the Christian Church. Pope Leo XIII., in an encyclical issued from the Vatican in November, 1901 A.D., said:

> "God alone is life. All other things partake of life, but are not life. Christ, from all eternity and by his very nature, is 'the Life,' just as He is the Truth, because He is God of God. From Him, as from its most sacred source, all life pervades and ever will pervade creation. Whatever is, is by Him; whatever lives, lives by Him. For 'by the Word all things were made; and without Him was made nothing that was made.'"

The same view of the origin of life and the great distinction between divine and natural, or secondary, causes was proclaimed in Rome nearly twenty centuries before this encyclical from our contemporary Pontifex Maximus, and under cir-

* *Paradise Lost*, xii. 430.

cumstances which lend a peculiar interest to it. The world is indebted to Cicero for the record of it, and to Macrobius for finding it after it had been supposed, for some fifteen centuries, to be irrevocably lost. I refer to the extraordinary vision attributed to Publius Cornelius Scipio, the second Scipio Africanus, while he was the military tribune in Africa and the guest of Prince Massanissa.

The night after his arrival, and after much talk about politics and government, but mostly of his ancestor, known as the first Africanus, Scipio retired to rest, and, as he said, "A sleep sounder than ordinary came over me." In his sleep he represents Africanus the elder to have presented himself, and to have predicted many things, favorable and menacing, to his descendant.

"Upon your single person," said Africanus, "the preservation of your country will depend; and, in short, it is your part, as dictator, to settle the government, if you can but escape the impious hands of your kinsmen. . . .

"But that you may be more earnest in the defence of your country, know from me that a certain place in heaven, where they are to enjoy an endless duration of happiness, is assigned to all who have preserved, or assisted, or improved their country. For there is nothing which takes place on earth more acceptable to that Supreme Deity who governs all this world than those councils and assemblies of men bound together by law which are termed states; the governors and preservers of these go hence, and hither do they return."

"Here," says Scipio, "frightened as I was, not so much from the dread of death as of the treachery of my friends, I asked him whether my father Paulus and others whom we thought to be dead were yet alive. '*To be sure they are alive,*' replied Africanus, '*for they have escaped from the fetters of the body as from a prison.* That which you call your life is really death. But behold your father Paulus approaching you.' No sooner did I see him," says Scipio, "than I poured forth a flood of tears; but he, embracing and kissing me, forbade me to weep. And when, having suppressed my tears, I began first to speak, 'Why,' said I, 'thou most sacred and excellent father, *since this is life,* as I hear Africanus affirm, *why do I tarry on earth,* and not hasten to come to you?'

"'Not so, my son,' he replied. 'Unless that God whose temple is all this which you behold shall free you from this imprisonment in the body you can have no admission to this place; for men have been created under this condition, that they should keep that globe which you see in the middle of this temple, and which is called the earth. And a soul has been supplied to them from those eternal fires which you call constellations and stars, and which, being globular and round, are animated with divine spirit, and complete their cycles and revolutions with amazing rapidity. Therefore you, my Publius, and all good men, must preserve your souls in the keeping of your bodies; nor without the order of that Being who bestowed them upon you, are you to depart from mundane life, lest you seem to desert the duty of a man, which has been assigned you by God. Therefore, Scipio, like your grandfather here, and me, who begot you, cultivate justice and piety, which, while it should be great towards your parents and relations, should be greatest towards your country. Such a life is the path to heaven and the assembly of those who have lived before, and who, having been released from their bodies, inhabit that place which thou beholdest.'"

"Truly, O Africanus," said the junior Scipio, "since the path to heaven lies open to those who have deserved well of their country, though from my childhood I have ever trod in your and my father's footsteps without disgracing your glory, yet now, with so noble a prize set before me, I shall strive with much more diligence.

"'Do so strive,' replied he, 'and *do not consider yourself, but your body, to be mortal. For you are not the being which this corporeal figure evinces; but the soul of every man is the man, and not that form which may be pointed at with a finger. Know, therefore, that you are a divine person. Since it is divinity that has consciousness, sensation, memory, and foresight—that governs, regulates, and moves that body over which it has been appointed, just as the Supreme Deity rules this world; and in like manner, as an eternal God guides this world, which in some respects is perishable, so an eternal spirit animates your frail body.*

"'For that which is ever moving is eternal. Now, that which communicates to another object a motion which it received elsewhere must necessarily cease to live as soon as its motion is at an end. Thus the being which is self-motive is the only being that is eternal, because it never is abandoned by its own properties, neither is this self-motion ever at an end; nay, this is the fountain, this is the beginning of motion to all things that are thus subjects of motion.

"'Since, therefore, it is plain that whatever is self-motive must be eternal, who can deny that this natural property is bestowed upon our minds? For everything that is moved by a foreign impulse is inanimate, but that which is animate is impelled by an inward and peculiar principle of motion; and in that consists the nature and property of the soul. Now, if it alone of all things is self-motive, assuredly it never was originated, and is eternal. Do thou, therefore, employ it in the noblest of pursuits, and the noblest of cares are those for the safety of thy country.'

"He vanished, and I awoke from my sleep."

This story comes to us as a dream. Whether a dream, a vision, or a meditation, science knows nothing and can presume nothing in conflict with this pagan's view either of life or death.

We absolutely know nothing of life which warrants us in attributing to it perishability; nor have we any reason to presume that with the change called death anything perishes, or that anything more has really occurred than a separation of the tenant from his habitation—of the soul from its material prison. Neither have we more reason to suppose that the spirit, or soul, has become less a soul, less an individual life, than that the matter with which it was clothed has been diminished in quantity by the separation. The destructibility of matter was, until comparatively recent times, just as popular a belief, and even more universally prevalent than is now that of the extinction of life when the soul leaves the body. Nor can science produce any evidence that the one belief was any more fallacious than the other. We are sent into this world and invested with material garments in order that we may be qualified to study and comprehend divine laws. The phenomenal world into which we are born is a kind of kindergarten where those divine laws are illustrated and made intelligible to our undeveloped and limited intelligence, through the operations of what we call Nature. It is a stage in our education when the phenomenal world is a necessity to us, as the hornbook and black-board are to school-children. When we have learned all the lessons in this kindergarten by which we are likely to profit we leave that school; and in leaving it, we assume the larger liberty of that higher life where time and space only signify differences in moral conditions; where, as in this life, we will seek the association and companionship of those with whom we shall then have most affinity.

All these, I say, are presumptions; and the burden of proof lies upon those who would undertake to maintain the contrary in any of these particulars.

Now, after we have shaken off this mortal coil and entered the world of spirits, in what respect does our condition differ from that of sleep? In both, our consciousness of this phenomenal world —of the kindergarten—has been entirely suspended. It is true that from sleep we awaken, sooner or later, to a consciousness of our incorporate limitations, while from death we do not awake. But is the difference any more than this—that in one case our carriage is left standing at the door to take us back again, while in the other we have no *animus revertendi?* Having reached home, we have no further use for our carriage and it is dismissed.

Nay, what reason have we for doubting that during our sleep we are in substantially the same society and surrounded by similar, if not the same, influences as we should be were we never again to awake? We cannot conceive that the abandonment of our earthly habitation, the laying aside of our garments, the deliverance from our prison, has deprived us of any of the qualities or attributes which constituted our being, except upon the theory of utter extinction by the separation. The spirit, or soul, inhabits the body, but is no more a part of it than the heat generated in a furnace is a part of the furnace or the light in our chamber is a part of the chamber. The inhabitants of the spiritual world are presumed to know nothing of the limitations of time or space. There is no manifest reason, therefore, why we should not always be accessible to and in intercourse with them, unless when too preoccupied by the distractions of our environment in the phenomenal world; nor for presuming that our *post-mortem* life will differ from our condition while sleeping, except that one is for a time and the other for eternity. As the spirit during sleep is presumptively as free as it ever will be from all the restrictions of sense, what reason is there for doubting that we enter at once into a life and a society substantially the same as that awaiting us when we enter into "the sleep that knows no waking"?

This presumption is strengthened by the fact that we can bring back no more information of what occurs to us in our temporary sleeps than we can from the spiritual world when we shall sleep with our fathers.

During our sleep we have no more power over anything in this phenomenal world than, while we are awake, we have over the spiritual world;

and yet, while asleep, we retain, in full activity, all the powers to act upon the world about us, save only the power or inclination to exert them. While this condition continues, what other or greater change could be wrought in us by death?

When we reflect upon the extraordinary change, psychological and physical, which we experience after a night's sound sleep, by what theory can that change be so satisfactorily and so rationally explained as to suppose that we have been temporarily in association with those who have preceded us to the spirit land? What is there improbable in this? What more entirely consistent with divine goodness? What so admirably, what so exclusively adapted to work the change which in the morning we realize has been worked in us during our slumbering? How very much more probable this, than that one-third of each day of our lives is permitted to go to waste, for which there is no imaginable explanation better than that a Creator, of infinite wisdom, could not fashion us in his image in any way that did not involve that waste—an absurd presumption.

While in a swoon or in immediate peril of drowning, as in some other cases of temporarily suspended action of the heart and lungs, persons have remained for hours, and even weeks, without any consciousness of the phenomenal life. During this suspended consciousness it is difficult to imagine any psychological difference between their condition and death.

The evidence is practically unanimous that while in a swoon or while near drowning, one's experience, instead of being painful, is altogether agreeable, even blissful, and entirely free from the concern and anxiety with which the prospect of death is ordinarily contemplated when awake.

An impressive illustration of what the death of the natural body means comes to us through the following Persian story, abridged from Sir Edwin Arnold's *Light of Asia:*

"DEATH OF ABDALLAH

"Faithful friends, it lies, I know,
Pale and white, and cold as snow;
And ye say, 'Abdallah's dead,'
Weeping at the feet and head.
I can see your falling tears,
I can hear your sighs and prayers;
Yet I smile and whisper this:
'*I* am not the thing you kiss!
Cease your tears and let it lie;
It *was* mine—it is not I.'

"Sweet friends, what the women lave
For the last sleep of the grave
Is the hut that I am quitting,
Is the garment no more fitting,
Is the cage from which at last,
Like a bird, my soul has passed.
Love the inmate, not the room;
The wearer, not the garb—the plume
Of the eagle, not the bars
That keep him from the splendid stars.

"Loving friends, oh, rise and dry
Straightway every weeping eye;
What ye lift upon the bier
Is not worth one single tear.
'Tis an empty sea-shell—one
Out of which the pearl is gone.
The shell is broken, it lies there;
The pearl, the *all*, the *soul* is here."

If this resemblance of sleep to death should seem chimerical to any, I have only to say that the teachings of the Bible on that subject must seem equally so. In that sacred record death and sleep are frequently—I might almost say constantly—used as equivalents.

Among the many marvels by which the death of Jesus on the cross was signalized, "the tombs were opened and many bodies of the saints that had *fallen asleep* were raised." *

In the first letter of Paul to the Corinthians he says:

"For I delivered unto you first of all that which also I received, how that Christ died for our sins according to the scriptures; and that he was buried; and that he hath been raised on the third day according to the scriptures; and that he appeared to Cephas; then to the twelve; then he appeared to five hundred brethren at once, of whom the greater part remain until now, but *some are fallen asleep.*" †

In the same letter Paul says:

* I Corinthians 15-20. † I Corinthians xv. 3-7.

"For if the dead are not raised, neither hath Christ been raised: and if Christ hath not been raised, your faith is vain; you are yet in your sins. Then they which are *fallen asleep* in Christ have perished. If in this life only we have hoped in Christ, we are of all most pitiable. But now hath Christ been raised from the dead, the first-fruits of them that *are asleep.*"

When Stephen was stoned to death for his loyalty to Jesus, he is reported to have kneeled down and cried with a loud voice, "Lord, lay not this to their charge. And when he had said this *he fell asleep.*"* We have no other authority for saying that he died.

Paul, in the thirteenth verse of the fourth chapter of his letter to the Thessalonians, says:

"But we would not have you ignorant, brethren, concerning them that *fall asleep;* that ye sorrow not, even as the rest, which have no hope. For if we believe that Jesus died and rose again, even so them also that are *fallen asleep* in Jesus will God bring with him."

Also, in the ninth verse of the fifth chapter of his letter to the Thessalonians, he says:

"For God appointed us not unto wrath, but unto the obtaining of salvation through our Lord Jesus Christ, who died for us, that, *whether we wake or sleep, we should live together with him.*"

"Knowing this first that there shall come in the last days scoffers walking after their own lusts, and

* Acts vii. 60.

saying, Where is the promise of his coming? for since the fathers *fell asleep*, all things continue as from the beginning of the creation." *

"David, after he had in his own generation served the counsel of God, *fell on sleep* and was laid unto his fathers."†

When the sisters of Lazarus sought Jesus, to tell Him that their brother was dead, He replied to them: "Our friend Lazarus sleepeth; but I go that I may awake him out of sleep." Then said his disciples: "If he sleep he shall do well"; howbeit Jesus spoke of his death. But they thought He had spoken of taking rest in sleep. Then said Jesus unto them, "Lazarus is dead."

Here we find Jesus calling the separation of the soul from the material body, which the disciples termed death, sleep; and it was not till the disciples showed that they misunderstood Him that He said, "Lazarus is dead."

The brethren of Lazarus said he was dead; Jesus said he slept. Did not both tell the truth?

When the prophet Elisha learned that the child of the Shunammite woman was dead he gave his servant Gehazi his staff and directed him to go and lay it upon the child. He did so, but was obliged to report to Elisha that "there was neither voice nor hearing. *The child is not awaked.*"

Elisha then came and found "the child was dead and laid upon his bed." He went in, shut to the

* 2 Peter iii. 3.

† Acts xiii. 36.

door, excluding all but the boy and himself and prayed unto the Lord. Then, after embracing him, "the flesh of the child waxed warm." Presently he sent for the mother and said to her, "Take up thy son."

Here the child had been dead. But all life comes from the Lord, and, in answer to the prophet's prayer, his body was warmed into life again; or, to use Gehazi's expression, was "awaked." *

The daughter of Jairus was given up for dead by her family. "Why make ye a tumult, and weep?" said Jesus, when He arrived, in response to a message from the father. "The child is not dead, but *sleepeth*. And they laughed him to scorn. But he, having put them all forth, taketh the father of the child and her mother and them that were with him, and goeth in where the child was. And taking the child by the hand, he saith unto her, Talitha cumi; which is, being interpreted, Damsel, I say unto thee, Arise. And straightway the damsel rose up, and walked; for she was twelve years old." †

Again in 1 Kings i. 21:

> "Otherwise it shall come to pass, when my lord the king *shall sleep with his fathers*, that I and my son Solomon shall be counted offenders."

* 2 Kings iv. 30–37.

† Mark v. 39; see also Acts ix. 10; xii. 6; Canticles v. 2; Hosea xii. 10; Jeremiah xxxi. 26; John xi. 11.

In the thirty-ninth verse of the fifty-first chapter of Jeremiah we read:

> "When they are heated, I will make their feast; and I will make them drunken, that they may rejoice, and sleep a perpetual sleep, and not wake, saith the Lord."

Secular and profane authority help to show how universally the conditions of sleep and death were assimilated in the popular mind throughout the ages.

It was the common belief of the ancient philosophers of Greece and Rome that the causes of sleep and death were the same. A place was assigned them in their Pantheon as brothers. Sleep was regarded both by the Epicureans and the Stoics, as well as by Plato, as death, followed by a resurrection. "Latet meus oppressa somno," says Lactantius, "tanquam ignis obducto cinere sopitus, quem si paulatim commoveris, rursus ardescit et quasi evigilabat."

Lucretius illustrates the same idea by the same metaphor: *

> "cinere ut multa latet obrutus ignis,
> Unde reconflari sensus per membra repente
> Possit, ut ex igni Cæco consurgere flamma."

Pausanias, describing the inscriptions on a chest, or cypsela, says:

> "On the other side of the chest, beginning from the

* *De Rerum Natura*, liber iv.

left hand, you will see a woman holding a white boy who is asleep, in her right hand, but in her left hand a black boy, who is likewise asleep and whose feet are distorted. The inscriptions signify—though you might infer without them—that these boys are Death and Sleep and that the Woman who is their nurse is Night." *

So when in the *Iliad* the large-eyed Juno remonstrated with the "dread Son of Saturn" for wishing to deliver Sarpedon

"from the common lot
Of death, a mortal doomed long since by fate,"

she finally suggested an alternative which was embraced:

"Yet if he be
So dear to thee and thou dost pity him,
Let him in mortal combat be o'ercome
By Menætiades, and when the breath
Of life has left his frame, give thou command
To Death and Gentle Sleep to bear him hence
To the broad realm of Lycia. There his friends
And brethren shall perform the funeral rites;
There shall they build him up a tomb and rear
A column—honors that become the dead." †

After Sarpedon had been slain by Patroclus, the Cloud-Compeller spake to Phœbus thus:

"Go now beloved Phœbus, and withdraw
Sarpedon from the weapons of his foes;

* *Pausanias*, book v. ch. 18.
† Homer's *Iliad*, Bryant's translation, book xvi. 565–575.

Cleanse him from the dark blood and bear him thence,
And lave him in the river-stream, and shed
Ambrosia o'er him. Clothe him then in robes
Of heaven, consigning him *to Sleep and Death,*
Twin brothers, and swift bearers of the dead;
And they shall lay him in Lycia's fields,
That broad and opulent realm—" etc.

Apollo instantly obeyed his father, sought the field of battle, bore off Sarpedon,

"And laved him in the river-stream and shed
Ambrosia o'er him. Then in robes of heaven
He clothed him, giving him to Sleep and Death,
Twin brothers and swift bearers of the dead,
And they, with speed conveying it, laid down
The corpse in Lycia's broad and opulent realm." *

Here Death and Sleep are twice designated as brothers and a third time are sent together on the same errand, implying functional equality.

Of the Golden Age, or Edenic period, Hesiod, the father of Greek poetry, said:

"As gods they lived, void of care, apart from labors and trouble; nor was wretched old age impending, and they died as if *overcome by sleep.*"

Xenophon, as quoted by Cicero, represents Cyrus, King of Persia, saying to his children on his death-bed:

"Do not believe, my dear children, that when I shall

* Homer's *Iliad*, Bryant's translation, book xvi. 833–853.

have quitted you I shall be nowhere and no more (*nunquam aut nullum fore*). While I was with you you did not see my soul; you only comprehended by my actions that this body was animated by one. I have never been able to persuade myself that souls that live while in mortal bodies, when they leave them die. I cannot believe that they lose all intelligence in quitting bodies that are essentially destitute of intelligence. When death disunites the human frame, we clearly see what becomes of its material parts; they apparently return to the several elements out of which they were composed; but the soul continues to remain invisible, both while present in the body and when it leaves it.

"You know, my children, that *nothing more resembles death than sleep;* and the sleep of souls chiefly proclaims their divinity, for many of them foresee the future and show what they will become when they shall be freed from the prison of the body." *

Sir Thomas Brown saw so little difference between sleep and death that he dared not lie down in his bed at night without saying his prayers and having a colloquy with God. He says:

"We are somewhat more than ourselves in our sleep, and the slumber of the body seems to be but the waking of the soul. It is the litigation of sense, but the liberty of reason, and our waking conceptions do not match the fancies of our sleeps. I am no way facetious nor disposed for the mirth and galliardize of company. Yet in one dream I can compose a whole comedy, behold the action, apprehend the jests, and laugh myself

* Cicero, *De Senectute*, ch. xxii.

awake at the conceits thereof. Were my memory as faithful as my reason is then fruitful, I would never study but in my dreams, and this time also would I choose for my devotions; but our grosser memories have then so little hold of our abstracted understandings that they forget the story, and can only relate to our awaked souls a confused and broken tale of that that hath passed.

. . . .

"Thus it is sometimes observed that men sometimes upon the hour of their departure do speak and reason above themselves; for then the soul, beginning to be freed from the ligaments of the body, begins to reason like herself and to discourse in a strain above mortality.

"We term sleep a death, and yet it is waking that kills us and destroys those spirits that are the house of life. *It is indeed a part of life that best expresses death.*

. . . .

"It is that death by which we may be said literally to die daily—a death which Adam died before his mortality; a death whereby we live a middle and moderating point between life and death; in fine, so like death, I dare not trust it without my prayers and a half adieu unto the world, and take my farewell in a colloquy with God." *

We have from the same distinguished physician the following lines, in which the identity of the states of sleep and death is, if possible, more distinctly asserted: †

* Sir Thomas Brown, b. 1605, d. 1682. *Religio Medici*, p. 131.

† Evening Hymn, by Sir Thomas Brown.

Sleep is a death; O make me try,
By sleeping, what it is to die;
And as gently lay my head
On my grave, as now my bed.
Howe'er I rest, great God, let me
Awake again at least with Thee.
And thus assured, behold I lie,
Securely, or to wake or die.
These are my drowsy days; in vain
I do now wake to sleep again:
O come that hour, when I shall never
Sleep again, but wake forever."

When these verses were written, Sir Thomas might have had in his mind the following lines of Heinrich Meibon, an Austrian poet-laureate, who died when Brown was but twenty years old:

" Alma quies optata veni; nam sic sine vita
Vivere quam suave est. sic sine morte mori." *

Henry Vaughan, the precursor of Wordsworth as the interpreter of the mystical and symbolical aspects of nature, in his verses entitled "The Morning Watch," has the following lines, quoted in the *Life and Times of Thomas Kettlewell,* by Francis Lee:

" Prayer is
The world in tune,
A Spirit Voice
And Vocall joyes,

* Come, refreshing sleep, we pray;
For without life how sweet to live;
Thus without death to die.

Whose Echo is heaven's blisse.
O let me climbe
When I lye down. The pious soul by nighte
Is like a clouded starre, whose beames, though said
To shed their light
Under some cloud,
Yet are above,
And shine and move
Beyond that mystic shroud.
So in my bed,
That curtained grave, though sleep like ashes hide
My lamp and life, both shall in Thee abide."

CHAPTER XI

"Whosoever shall say, Thou fool, shall be in danger of the hell of fire."

IF I have been so fortunate as to carry any of my readers with me thus far, I hope they will be prepared to concede that any, even a partial, suspension of our consciousness weakens to a corresponding extent our bondage to the phenomenal or material world; and, on the other hand, that the man who allows himself to be too long and too much interested in any worldly subject or employ sooner or later is liable to unbalance his mind and become at first a crank, and ultimately a lunatic.

And this invites a consideration of some of the effects of the occasional interruptions of any current of thought or diversion of our mind from worldly interests that are becoming so absorbing as to threaten our spiritual freedom.

It rarely occurs to any of us to consider how numerous and providential these interruptions are, and how felicitously they supplement the divinely appointed offices of sleep.

How many of our household and family cares, how many of the exactions of children, of society, and of the countless interruptions which constitute the woof in the warp of every man's life, are providentially thrust upon us like sleep, weakening the undue hold of the world upon our affections. We treat many of them as trifles; at more of them we murmur and often rudely complain, frequently not shrinking from suicide, never thinking that they not only may be, but are, messengers of mercy—supplementary Sabbaths of divine appointment.

It is a prevailing impression, intrenched behind numerous proverbs, that all our time during our waking hours not employed in the prosecution of what may be generically called business is wasted, that a man who is not working for some worldly purpose to some worldly end is an idle man, and that an idle man is a drone, of no use to society, and, if our race were as wise as the bee, we would expel him from it.

This, as a rule, is a great delusion. The man who "sits silent"—to use a phrase of the Society of Friends—may certainly have one great advantage of the busy man, for if not making the best possible use of his time, he is less likely to be the slave of this-worldliness than the busy man. His mind is more open and accessible to spiritual impressions, or, if you please, less liable to be preoccupied with worldly and selfish matters, than the more worldly man.

It strikes most of us as a very original and surprising conceit of Milton, though it ought to be with all of us the perfection of commonplace, that

> "He also serves who only stands and waits."

But how few there are in this driving age who really take any time to "wait," to listen to the still, small voices, to reflect, to dream. Instead of thinking themselves, they get the people of the press, the forum, or the market-place, to think for them.

Nothing is spiritually more impoverishing for a man than to allow himself no time for dreaming; to feed habitually, if not exclusively, upon other people's thoughts, and rarely or never upon his own. In that respect children ordinarily have the advantage of adults, the world not having yet reduced their imaginations to its stupefying bondage. In the language of the greatest of Roman satirists, in his quest of the means of living man forgets the ends of life. He fancies himself the source and proprietor of the power he wields, and that the "kingdom, power, and glory" is not his Creator's but his own.

Joseph was called by his brethren a dreamer. These brethren were no mean types of modern society, which is constantly laying violent hands upon our faculties for dreaming, for waiting, and for thinking. Of the sisters of Lazarus, the modern world sympathizes most with Martha, who was careful and troubled about her housekeeping; but it was not without a good reason that Jesus commended Mary.

We never know why it rains just as we are setting out on a picnic; why a child falls sick as we are about to embark on a journey; why the news of a death in the family prevents our going to a dinner or a ball on which we had set our heart; why the bank failed in which we had left our money. Still less do we know from what evils they may have shielded us. We should never forget that none of our disappointments are fortuitous, nor that one of the most obvious and constant advantages we derive from them is the same as that for which we are in a larger degree indebted to sleep.

Even sickness, the most familiar and universal deranger of the plans of men, is in most cases the result of too much this-worldliness, and also the most effective cure of it.

In taking leave of his pupils at the College of Charlemagne in 1841, in consequence of failing health, Jouffroy said: "Disease is certainly a grace with which God favors us—a sort of spiritual retreat which He provides us, that we may recognize ourselves, find ourselves, and restore to our sight the true view of things."

One of the greatest problems with which psychologists have been puzzled has been to ascertain the moral condition of an insane person — that is, of a person who attaches undue and disproportionate value to privileges and distinctions of this world; whether it is, morally, a progressive, a passive, or a retrogressive state; and, if not progressive, how such a state is to be reconciled with that love of God which is supposed to be always operative over all his works.

When Jesus was told that his father and mother were without, waiting for Him, He replied: "Know ye not that I must be about my father's business?" Jesus is always about his Father's business; always knocking at every man's door, trying to arrest his attention, and waiting for an invitation to come in and sup with him. He cannot be presumed ever to leave one of his children in a condition by night or by day when the process of their regeneration, which is the end and final purpose of their creation, cannot progress.

When we cease to be susceptible of spiritual growth in this world our life in it necessarily ceases.

God cannot be suspected of providing life and a terrestrial environment in this world for any except to educate them for a higher life. A contrary supposition must assume that the Omnipotent and the Omniscient could permit any waste of his energy. That is not supposable. Hence we are forced to the conclusion that if lunatics and idiots have reached their spiritual growth, and are capable of no more spiritual improvement, it is as idle to suppose that their Creator would continue to supply them with his breath of life as that He should continue to supply sap to a dead tree. No one's days can be presumed to continue an hour longer than he possesses the ability to choose between good and evil and is capable of being fashioned into a less imperfect image of his Creator. It is for that, and that only, we are put into this world; and there is no power willing and competent to keep us here a moment after that ability fails us. We are forced, therefore—at least, every Christian is forced—by a logical necessity to the conclusion that divine grace is just as operative with the wildest demoniac and the most helpless idiot as it ever was with the apostles Paul and John.

The most conspicuous feature of insanity is the more or less complete obscuration of the victim's mental appreciation of one or more of the most familiar laws which govern the phenomenal world. He seems to live—a part of the time, at least—in quite a different world from that in which sane people about him are living. He even becomes to himself an entirely different person or object from what he appears to be to others.

Charles Lamb has told us that during the early part of his life he was constrained to retire to a lunatic asylum, where he was detained for several months. In a letter to his friend Coleridge, written a few years after his recovery, he said:

"At some future time I will amuse you with an account, as full as my memory will permit, of the strange turn my frenzy took. I look back upon it at times with a gloomy kind of envy; for while it lasted I had many, many hours of pure happiness. Dream not, Coleridge, of having tasted all the grandeur and wildness of fancy till you have gone mad."

Is not a lunatic in much the same condition as a person dreaming, partially sensible of the phenomenal world and partially insensible of it? He will talk coherently for a time about some things, incoherently about others at other times, but in a way that shows his mind is only partially alive to the relations of this world; so that what he says or does may be as inconsequential as what we ordinarily remember of a dream. Yet his mind is obviously quite as active when his talk is incoherent as when it is coherent. May he not be as sane as any other man appears to be in a dream? May not his attention be divided between the two worlds which, like the dreamer, he seems to inhabit? May not the society in which he finds himself at times when to others he seems insane be as real as any other?—and may not agencies be at work as constantly for his regeneration as for any other of God's children?

Insanity has many causes, but the kind of insanity with which we are most familiar results from a disproportionate activity of some psychic qualities: ambition, avarice, vanity, an undue estimate of our importance in the regulation of the world, which, whether inherited or acquired, induce a disproportionate activity of certain emotions, which gradually, like all our appetites, grow by what they feed on, until they overmaster the reason and disqualify one for taking the precautions and avoiding the practices and habits for which they lust.

One of the first evidences of this loss of balance is usually insomnia. Most suicides are, directly or indirectly, attributable to the same cause. But where, I may be asked, are the evidences of divine love in such dispensations? That question may be most conveniently answered by asking another: What would be the consequences of allowing a person whose vanity or ambition, or other inordinate appetite, led him to the indulgence of such excesses for its gratification, if its progress were not arrested by the impairment of other faculties that go to make up the balance of a healthy character, but over which his reason, without being seriously impaired, had ceased to have control? He would evidently become by degrees a monster—such a monster as to be capable of any crime, and entirely inaccessible to any rectifying spiritual influences.

We are all of us more or less familiar with the perils we have providentially escaped through our disappointments and reverses in life. Are we not all in a certain sense like lunatics—victims of a more or less unbalanced mind? And is not the work of spiritual regeneration simply the effort, through divine aid, to restore that balance? And in the proportion that a lunatic is disqualified to take a sensible and rational interest in the phenomenal world, may he not to that extent be made accessible to regenerating influences of a similar character with those we have supposed to be operative during the suspension of our consciousness in sleep?

No one has ever ventured to sneer at Dryden's remark that "Great wits are sure to madness near allied." One can easily be persuaded by a reference to the biographies of men of genius that this poet's words deserve to be taken quite seriously.

Lucretius, the greatest poet of ancient Italy, and Tasso, the greatest poet of modern Italy, both wrote the works to which they owe their fame with posterity during the interruptions of frequent attacks of lunacy. The former is said by St. Jerome to have died by his own hand at the comparatively early age of forty-four, leaving unfinished that greatest monument of Roman literary genius, the *De Rerum Natura*.

Tasso, like Socrates, believed he had a familiar spirit, or genius, that was pleased to talk with him, and from whom he learned things never before heard of.

Cæsar was an epileptic and subject to cerebral disorder. Charles V. was an epileptic; he took refuge from his throne in a monastery, where he had his own funeral rites celebrated in his presence—two of the many evidences he gave of an unbalanced mind. His mother was insane, and his grandfather, Ferdinand of Aragon, died, at the comparatively early age of sixty-two, in a state of profound melancholia.

Linnæus died in a state of senile dementia.

Raphael had more or less of the suicidal mania.

Pascal could not bear to see his father and mother together, though pleased to see either separately; neither could he see water without transports of vexation.

Walter Scott, during the latter portion of his life, had visions betokening an unbalanced mind.

Michael Angelo attempted to starve himself to death, and was only saved by the interference of his physician.

Richelieu had attacks of insanity. His elder brother committed suicide, and his sister also was insane.

Descartes imagined himself followed by an invisible person urging him to pursue his investigations in search of the Absolute.

Goethe fancied he saw the image of himself coming to meet him.

Cromwell had violent attacks of melancholia, and a sickly, neuropathic constitution from his birth.

Jean Jacques Rousseau suffered all his life from an unbalanced mind, and not infrequently from attacks of acute delirium and maniacal excitation. He died from an apoplectic attack.

Mohammed was epileptic, and claimed to be

a messenger from God and to have had interviews with the Angel Gabriel.

Molière was a neuropath, and any delay or derangement of his plans would throw him into convulsions.

Mozart was subject to fainting fits before and during the composition of his famous "Requiem." He imagined messengers were sent to him to announce his end. He died at the early age of thirty-six of cerebral hydropsy.

Cuvier is said to have died of a disease of the nervous centres. He lost all his children by cerebral fever.

Condillac was a somnambulist.

Bossuet is known occasionally to have lost the faculty of speech, and even of understanding.

Madame de Staël died in a delirium said to have lasted several months. She had a nervous habit of rolling between her fingers small strips of paper, an ample supply of which was kept on her mantel-piece. She had a nervous fear of being cold in the tomb, and desired to be enveloped in furs before burial.

Swift from an early period of his life was queer, and "died at the top," a violent maniac. He was called the "Mad Parson."

Shelley suffered from somnambulism, disturbing dreams, and an excitable and impetuous temperament, which increased with age. He was called "Mad Shelley."

Samuel Johnson was a hypochondriac, had

hallucinations and convulsions, and was constantly apprehensive of insanity.

Southey wrote verses before he was eight years of age, and died an imbecile.

Cowper was attacked with melancholia at the age of twenty, from which he suffered for a year. It subsequently returned. He tells of attempts at suicide, and he would have hanged himself had not the rope broken from which he suspended himself.

Keats was subject to fits of despondency, and was so nervous that the glitter of the sun or the sight of a flower made him tremble.

Coleridge was a precocious child and had a morbid imagination. When thirty years of age he took to the use of opium.

Burns tells us that his constitution from the beginning "was blasted with a deep, incurable taint of melancholia which poisons my existence."

George Eliot was extremely sensitive to terror in the night, and remained "a quivering fear" throughout her whole life.

De Quincey, in consequence of general nervous irritability, took opium to excess.

Alfred de Musset had attacks which George Sand described as manifesting a nervous condition approaching delirium. He had a suicidal inclination. He had hallucinations which compelled him to ask his brother to assist him in distinguishing it from real things.

Carlyle showed extreme irritability, and spoke

of himself in his diary: "Nerves all inflamed and torn up, body and mind in a hag-ridden condition."

Bach and Handel were both very irritable, great sufferers from nervous troubles, and both died of apoplexy.

Newton in his latter years was subject to a melancholia which deprived him of all power of thought. In a letter to Locke he says that he "passed some months without having a consistency of mind."

Alexander the Great had from infancy neurosis of the muscles of the neck, and died at the age of thirty-two, exhibiting all the symptoms of acute delirium tremens. Both his parents were dissolute, and his brother was an idiot.

Lamartine was a crank, like his father before him.

William Pitt, Earl of Chatham, was descended from a family exhibiting many peculiarities and mental disproportions approaching alienation.

Pope was rickety and subject to hallucinations.

Lord Byron was scrofulous, rachitic, imagined he was visited by a ghost, which he attributed to the over-excitability of his brain. Lord Dudley did not disguise his conviction that Byron was insane.

Napoleon I. feared apoplexy and was subject to hallucinations.

There is no occasion to enlarge this list, as it

might be indefinitely. In the instances we have selected there is sufficient evidence that insanity probably is, and certainly may be, a providential interruption of degenerating and pernicious tendencies. Even with our short sight, these tendencies may be traced to an unequal and disproportioned interest in some of our worldly affairs and the consequent enfeeblement of others intended to be regulating or compensating faculties. But it is blasphemous to suppose that the class of men so conspicuous for their usefulness in the world, to whose unbalanced minds attention has just been called, were not to the last, as much as ever, the objects of God's uninterrupted and inexhaustible love and mercy. There is really no more reason for supposing there is such an interruption in the case of lunatics than there is for a like supposition in the case of those whose consciousness is suspended by sleep. The impairment of some of their faculties may have been rendered necessary to prevent their confirmation in evils to which they may have been prone, just as all of us are more or less withheld in our slumbers, and thus made amenable to spiritual influences to which otherwise they would have been inaccessible.

Let it not be supposed that the changes here referred to are physical or the results of morbid cerebration, as was so flippantly taught not many years ago by many eminent French physicians; for we have abundant medical authority to the contrary. "Frequent autopsies," says Chauvet,* "reveal no appreciable difference between the brain of a lunatic and a man of unimpaired mental integrity. Such is the affirmation of all conscientious physicians who have made a special study of mental maladies."

It is a medical aphorism as old at least as Hippocrates that a sufferer from a painful disease generally loses all consciousness of it on becoming deranged. A disorder of the mind replaces the disorder of the body. In illustration of this, De Bönnenhausen, on the authority of the chronicler Bulan, *Hist. Secr.* i. 12, quotes the following experience of the grandmother of Mirabeau:

"This *femme bigote,*" as he calls her, "eighty years of age and emaciated to a skeleton, was attacked, in consequence of a wrong treatment for the gout, with a furious nymphomania. From that moment she seemed to renew her youth; her monthly courses reappeared. This healthy period lasted for four years, but she rapidly sank and expired with the return of reason."

Here is a case of a person experiencing for a series of years an extraordinary rejuvenescence of strength and respite from pain by being to a considerable extent cut off from ordinary relations and communication with the phenomenal world. She was *bigote,* says De Bönnenhausen. Was

* *Nouveaux Principes de Philosophie Médicale,* par le Dr. N. M. Chauvet.

not Providence clearly dealing with this infirmity as it had once dealt with St. Paul's, by cutting off her relations with an environment which had developed that mental disease, and reducing her to a condition which protected her from its influence, substituting a love for others, though on the natural plane, in the place, perhaps, of a morbid self-righteousness?

When Jesus and his disciples came down from the Mount of Transfiguration there came a man who, kneeling down to Him, said, "Lord, have mercy on my son: for he is a lunatic and sore vexed: and oft-times he falleth into the fire, and oft into the water. And I brought him to thy disciples, and they could not cure him." We are told that "Jesus rebuked the devil, and he departed out of him; and the child was cured from that very hour."

While Jesus was in the borders of Tyre and Sidon, a Syrophœnician woman whose young daughter had an unclean spirit "besought him that he would cast forth the devil out of her daughter." For the faith exhibited by this mother, He said: "Go thy way; the devil is gone out of thy daughter. And when she was come to her house, she found the devil gone out and her daughter laid upon the bed." *

The man with an unclean spirit, who could not be bound even with a chain, and whom no

* Mark vii. 26–30.

man could tame, when *he saw Jesus*, ran and worshipped Him. Jesus bade the evil spirit come out of him, and the demoniac was left clothed and in his right mind. He then begged to remain with Jesus, but Jesus made a missionary of him, as later he did of Paul of Tarsus.*

Jesus may be seen by the feeble-minded to-day just as distinctly as when seen by this demoniac in Syria.

While we are permitted to assume that the insane and the idiotic, so far as they are detached from the phenomenal world, may be, to the same limited extent, in the condition of the sleeper and in a degree sharing the advantages which the condition of sleep is supposed to provide, it must not be inferred that any form or degree of insanity is in itself desirable, otherwise than as it tends to arrest spiritual tendencies of a more perilous character.

Insanity may be presumed to be in most cases the fruit of either deliberate or hereditary tendencies which conflict with divine order. The cases with which we are all of us most familiar are of persons who have become insane by overwork or by resorting to artificial means for superseding the demands of their constitution for sleep. As these excesses are commonly the results of inordinate ambition or vanity or greed, and when these spiritual infirmities reach a stage where

* Mark v. 2–20.

any voluntary arrest of them is hopeless, a merciful Providence may be presumed so to modify their relations with the phenomenal world as to prevent further spiritual degeneration. In some cases the ministrations of Jesus warrant us in thinking that the work of regeneration is allowed to progress. All that can be said with confidence of the influence of insanity is that in detaching its victim from habitual this-worldliness it so far resembles the operation of sleep, and is a real and usually an unappreciated evidence of divine mercy. A French investigator has reached the conclusion that the brains of military men give out most quickly; that out of every 100,000 men of the army or naval profession, 199 are hopeless lunatics. Of the liberal professions, artists are the first to succumb to the brain-strain. Is there nothing in the inspirations and aspirations of these pursuits to explain these results?

CHAPTER XII

Why we are not permitted to be conscious of the experiences of the soul in sleep—How we should cultivate sleep—Drugs hostile to sleep—Count Tolstoi on alcoholic stimulants—All virtues favor sleep; all vices discourage it.

IF by the immutable laws of our being the hours consecrated to sleep are, as I have attempted to show, of such vital importance to our spiritual development, the ordering of our life, so far as it may affect our sleep, assumes a corresponding importance. No argument is needed to prove that we should make it our study to avoid as far as possible everything calculated to interfere in the slightest degree with its completeness. All such disturbances may be presumed to come from our phenomenal life, and so far, at any rate, as they do, they impair the completeness of our isolation from the world and its works, and violate the sacred mysteries to which it is the presumptive purpose of sleep to admit the soul —our real self—for the reception of such spiritual instruction as we may be qualified to assimilate, without bringing away with us any knowledge that can interfere with the freedom of our will or with our personal responsibility for what we may do in our waking hours.

I say without bringing away anything that would interfere with the freedom of our will, because what goes on within us in our sleep is as sacred a mystery as any of the mysteries of our eternal sleep; nor is it difficult to divine a sufficient purpose for that mystery. If we were as conscious of our sleeping as of our waking life, and if our external memory, as Swedenborg calls it, could bring away our experiences while in that state; could reveal to us the treasures of our interior memory, it would interfere with our freedom in precisely the same way and degree as if we could foresee the influence of our acts and plans of yesterday upon all the future stages of our existence. Such knowledge would be fatal to our spiritual growth and to the freedom of our will, through which only righteousness thrives; would give place to a blind, senseless fatalism.

We may speculate about the purposes of Providence as revealed in the sequence of the events of our daily life, but we know nothing, and think little, if anything, of them when they occur. It is only long after their occurrence that we begin to realize how much more profoundly they affected the tenor of our lives than we had suspected they would; from what perils we had been protected by what we regarded as grievous disappointments; from what temptations, which we could never have resisted, we had been shielded by our ignorance, by our weaknesses, by discouragements, by poverty, by sickness, etc. If God in his providence makes us so blind to the consequence of what we do in our waking hours, the wisdom of which experience ultimately compels us not only to admit but to be thankful for, there is no reason to question the divine wisdom in concealing from us what it is trying to do for us in our sleep when the god of this world is disarmed and powerless.

It would be tedious to enumerate all the things done in what is called civilized society that, consciously and unconsciously, interfere with the quality and quantity of our sleep. A volume would not suffice for such a record. I may only speak of them by classes.

First in importance among these I would place what we take into our mouths under the name or disguise of nourishment. There is scarcely a table laid in all our broad land on which will not be found more or less of the enemies of wholesome sleep: condiments selected primarily to stimulate the appetite, but provoking to gluttony and animal indulgence, regardless of the divine purposes for which we were endowed with these appetites, and with power both to guide and control them. It is a fact worthy of the profoundest consideration that about everything we take into our mouths, not simply for our nourishment, but to provoke our appetites and for the sole pleasure of gratifying them, discourages sleep.

"If one wishes to make others do wrong," says Count Tolstoi,* "he alcoholizes them. They make soldiers drunk before sending them into battle. At the time of the assault of Sebastopol all the French soldiers were drunk. It is well known that robbers, brigands, and prostitutes cannot dispense with alcohol. All the world agrees that the consumption of these narcotics has for its object stifling the remorse of conscience; and yet, in cases where the use of these exhilarants does not result in assassination, theft, and violence, they are not condemned."

To the defence that a light exhilaration—that is to say, initial drunkenness, which is but a partial eclipse of the judgment—cannot produce very important consequences, the Count makes this clever reply:

"A famous Russian painter one day corrected a picture made by one of his pupils. He gave a few touches of his pencil here and there, but the result was such, nevertheless, that the pupil cried out, 'You made but two or three marks on my picture, and I find it completely changed.' The painter replied, 'Art does not begin but where marks scarcely perceptible produce great changes.' These remarks," he adds, "are remarkably just, not only in relation to art, but all the conditions of human life."

* Translated from an article published some years ago in the *Revue Rose*.

Dr. Franklin, in a letter written to a Miss on the art of procuring pleasant dreams, said:

> "In general, mankind, since the improvement of cookery, eat about twice as much as nature requires. Suppers are not bad, if we have not dined; but restless nights naturally follow hearty suppers after full dinners. Indeed, as there is a difference in constitutions, some rest well after these meals; it costs them only a frightful dream, and an apoplexy, after which they sleep till doomsday."

Among the antisoporifics, next in importance come the apothecaries' drug-poisons. Of these there are very few—I fear none—the direct or secondary action of which is not hostile to sleep. The uncorrupted tastes and instincts of the beasts of the field reject them all, as well in sickness as in health.

It is a curious illustration of the limitations of what we call civilization that the one art or science which we hedge about with the most arbitrary laws for the protection of its priesthood and ministrants, and which is relied upon to prevent or cure our diseases, should be the one organized professional body which practically employs few, if any, therapeutic agencies that do not impair, discourage, or prevent sleep, and to the same extent shorten life. If in the whole pharmacopœia of those who claim to be "the regular medical faculty" there is a single drug which is not a poison and which is not more or less actively hostile to sleep, it is one which is scarcely, if ever, used, except to impress the imagination rather than the disorder of the patient. Should any of my readers think this statement an exaggeration they will find little difficulty in ascertaining that it is not. The homœopathists are compelled by the fundamental law of their therapeutics to ascertain the effects of every drug by testing them upon persons in sound health. In that way they have stored up in their literature most of all that is known of the direct effects of all the drugs that have proved to be sufficiently reactionary for therapeutical purposes, which means all drugs in general use. The reader has only to turn to Jahr's *Manual of Medicine* or Herring's *Condensed Materia Medica* to satisfy himself of the insomniac influences which radiate from every apothecary's shop.*

* Here are a few drugs recorded by Jahr under a single initial letter, with the symptoms relating to sleep for which they are responsible:

Aconitum napellus—Sleeplessness from anxiety, with constant agitation and tossing; startings in sleep; anxious dreams with nightmare.

Agnus costus—Disturbed sleep, waking with a start.

Alumina—Nocturnal sleep too light; frequent waking in the night; nightmare; during the night anxiety, agitation, and tossing about.

Ambergris—Agitated sleep with anxious dreams; startings with fright.

Ammoniac—Sleep unquiet during the night; numerous and painful dreams.

Ammonia, carbonate of — Nightmare when falling

With drug-poisons should be classed nearly, if not quite, all fermented drinks—the most costly part of most people's diet who indulge in them at all—coffee, tea, tobacco, spices, and most of the constantly multiplying tonics and condiments of the table. All of them have a tendency, directly or indirectly, to discourage or impair sleep, and, as such, are *hostes humani generis*. Their interference with sleep, though perhaps the most serious, is very far from being their only pathogenetic influence.

The late Dr. Alonzo Clark, who for years stood quite at the head of his profession as a consulting physician in New York City, is quoted as au-

asleep; dreams of spectres, death, of vermin, and of quarrels.

Ammonium causticum—Disturbed sleep.

Ammonium muriaticum—Restlessness before midnight; many dreams, anxious, terrific, or lascivious; nocturnal sweat after midnight.

Anacardium orientale (Malacca bean)—Disturbed sleep in the night; anxious dreams, disgusting or horrible, with cries; lively dreams of projects, of fire, of diseases, of deaths, and of dangers.

Angustura bark—Sleep disturbed by frequent dreams.

Antimonium crudum—Waking with fright during the night; dreams, anxious, horrible, voluptuous, or painful, and full of quarrelling.

Arnica—Sleep full of anxious and terrible dreams and waking with starts and fright; dreams of death, of mutilated bodies; giddiness on waking.

Arsenicum—During sleep, startings with fright, groans; frequent dreams full of fears, threats, apprehensions.

Assafœtida—Sleep unrefreshing, with tossing and frequent waking.

Aurum—Restless sleep with anxious dreams.

thority for saying: "All curative agents, so called, are poisons, and, as a consequence, every dose diminishes the patient's vitality." I doubt whether this view of drugs would be seriously contested by any of his professional brethren of good standing.

The late venerable Professor Joseph M. Smith, M.D., said: "All medicines which enter the circulation poison the blood in the same manner as do the poisons that produce the disease. Drugs do not cure disease. Digitalis has hurried thousands to the grave. Prussic acid was once extensively used in the treatment of consumption, both in Europe and America, but its reputation is lost. Thousands of patients were treated with it, but not a case was benefited. On the contrary, hundreds were hurried to the grave."

Digitalis is regarded by old-school physicians as a specific for heart-failure. Here are its symptoms as recorded in Jahr's manual:

> Sleep—Drowsiness in the day and somnolency interrupted by convulsive vomiting; at night, half sleep with agitation; nocturnal sleep, interrupted by anxious dreams, with starts.

R. Clarke Newton, in his treatise on *Opium and Alcohol*, says:

> "Sleeplessness means not merely unrest, but starvation of the cerebrum. The only cause for regret in these cases is that the blunder should ever be committed of supposing that a stupefying drug which throws the brain into a condition that mimics and burlesques

sleep can do good. It is deceptive to give narcotics in a case of this type. The stupor simply masks the danger. Better far let the sleepless patient exhaust himself than stupefy him. Chloral bromide and the rest of the poisons that produce a semblance of sleep are so many snares in such cases. Sleeplessness is a malady of the most formidable character, but it is not to be treated by intoxicating the organ upon which the stress of the trouble falls. Suicide, which occurs at the very outset of derangement, and is apt to appear a sane act, is the logical issue of failure of nutrition that results from want of sleep."

It is a fact now recognized by the medical profession that the use of narcotics, fermented liquors, and other intoxicants by which the people of all nations seek pleasure—simple oblivion of the troubles of life or of its sorrows, of its chagrins or of destitution—produce temporarily precisely the condition in which a man finds himself in a dream. The faculty explain it by lesions, obstructions, disorganizations of tissues, cells, nerve centres, liver and kidneys, etc. These are physical changes incident to the use of these disorganizing agencies. In point of fact, it is these disorganizing agencies that produce the partial, sometimes temporary, sometimes chronic, insensibility to mental or physical troubles by impairing our consciousness of them, just as our consciousness of them is totally suspended in sleep and partially suspended in dreams when we have begun to awake. These dreams are sometimes prolonged, and result in what is commonly termed dementia.

Lasègue tells us that the alcoholic delirium is not a delirium, but a dream.* Max-Simon says: "The alcoholic patient commences his delirium in his dream during sleep and continues it on awaking, while other lunatics, melancholics, paralytics, maniacs, find in sleep a truce to their delirium." †

At first the dream of the alcoholic appears as a passing trouble and ceases on awakening. It is only a nightmare. After a while the dream is prolonged beyond the awakening, and it exteriorizes itself in a sort of tranquillized delirium. Finally, auto-intoxication reaches its maximum in that peculiar mental state described first by an eminent French physician as *mental confusion*. The recollection of the dream may survive the dream itself for some time, and become a sort of subacute delirium, to which Baillarger has given the name of *fixed ideas*.‡

While this similarity between dreams and a person intoxicated by narcotics, alcoholics, hashish, or any of the thousand drugs to which people have recourse for temporary alleviation of pain or sorrow, distress or depression of any kind, is

* Lasègue, *Archives Générales de Médecine*. 1881.

† Max-Simon, *Le Monde des Rêves*. Paris, 1882.

‡ Baillarger, "De l'Influence de l'État Intermédiaire à la Veille et au Sommeil sur la Production des Hallucinations." *Annales Médico-Psychologiques*. 1845.

so universally recognized by the medical faculty, it seems to have occurred to none of them that the remedy for relief in every case is precisely the same as that which is sought through sleep — to make us insensible to our troubles and forget the world in which they originate. Their similarity to dreams consists in the insensibility produced by these drugs—that is, the partial suspension of consciousness. What a deplorable fact it is that, instead of sleep, so large a proportion of the human race resort to these noxious substitutes for it! What a mercy that where the will is too weak to resist the temptation to resort to these substitutes, "the wisdom of their wise men shall perish, and the understanding of their prudent men shall be hid"!*

Then comes the strife for wealth, and power, and position among men; the undue accumulation of cares and responsibilities, the result in most cases of unbridled ambition, vanity, or greed.

It is the middle-aged and old who suffer most from this infirmity.

> "Care keeps his watch in every old man's eye,
> And where he lodges sleep can never lie;
> But where unbruised youth, with unstuffed brain,
> Doth crouch his limbs, there sleep doth reign."

Whenever a man has reached threescore-and-ten, and, in railway parlance, is started on the

* Isaiah xxix. 14.

down grade, he should study to simplify his life so as never to be required to draw upon his reserves, nor work under pressure, or with a conscious overdraft of nervous force. A neglect of this precaution is pretty certain to interfere with both the quantity and quality of our sleep, and sooner or later to compel a resort to stimulants of one kind or another, by which we borrow for the day the strength of to-morrow, thus speedily to become hopelessly indebted to nature, the most inexorable of creditors.

Speaking of reports, which but too frequently meet our eyes in the public prints, of men prominent in religious movements who have disgraced themselves and discredited the faith they professed by ignominious peculations, embezzlements, and frauds, the late Dr. A. P. Peabody, of Harvard University, said:

"We are not surprised that these instances have been placed and kept prominently before the community; for such cases are so rare as justly to arrest grave attention and excite emphatic comment. So far as we know, they are, all of them, cases in which there had been for a long period such an engrossment in multifarious, crowding, and perplexing business operations that the religious life was physically impossible, the quietness essential to devotion unattainable, supersensual themes of thought excluded by a necessity, self-imposed indeed, but imposed—there is reason to believe—before the first steps in the direction of overt guilt and shame. No Christian of sane mind will pretend or imagine that church-going with the inward ear closed and deafened, the form of Christian communion without the spirit of the cross, Sunday overlaid by the cares of the preceding and the forecast shadows of the coming week, are a moral specific; and many who call, and perhaps think, themselves Christians *are in intense need of precisely the lessons which these disasters among their own brotherhood may teach.*"

All the appetites, propensities, lusts, and passions which we cannot control are incidental to, and evidences of, our unregenerate nature; are the weaknesses of the flesh which it is the end and purpose of our probationary life on earth to subdue. It is a fact most important, early to learn and never to lose sight of, that all these appetites, propensities, and passions are unrelenting enemies of sleep. It is the most impressive illustration of the inflexible logic of Providence that as they all, if allowed free rein, tend to impair the health, blunt the senses one by one, diminish, and finally extinguish, the enjoyment they were designed to yield; they, in that way, like old age, are permitted to serve in a measure the purposes of sleep, in detaching man from the world by depriving him of the means of enjoying what he persists in abusing, and thus of "withdrawing him from his purpose, and in keeping him from the pit."

It would be well for every one to realize that all the virtues favor sleep and all the vices discourage it. In the gratification of our appetites it is our highest duty to respect the laws of our being which impose self-control. Whether we eat too much, or drink too much, or devote too large a portion of our time and strength to any employment or amusement, the first rebuke which nature administers for such intemperance is a change in the quantity or quality of our sleep; conscience, attended by the dragons of remorse, follows us to our chamber and tells us that sleep shall not refresh us until we repent of our excesses. In the degree in which we respect the laws of our being, which are the ordinances of our Creator, will be the sufficiency of our rest. In the degree that we disregard them will be its insufficiency.

The desire—nay, the necessity—for sleep should be regarded as a providential arrangement to induce us to cultivate the virtues most favorable to its enjoyment, just as hunger and thirst are the agents of Providence for teaching us to be frugal, industrious, and temperate, that they may be reasonably gratified.

If these things be true about sleep, they obviously impose duties upon the pulpit, upon the press, and upon all human society which are sadly neglected.

APPENDIX A

Ralph Waldo Emerson's estimate of Swedenborg:

". . . Emanuel Swedenborg, . . . who appears to his contemporaries a visionary, . . . no doubt led the most real life of any man then in the world; and now, when the royal and ducal Frederics . . . of that day have slid into oblivion, he begins to spread himself into the minds of thousands. As happens in great men, he seemed, by the variety and amount of his powers, to be a composition of several persons, like the giant fruits which are matured in gardens by the union of four or five single blossoms. . . . He was a scholar from a child. . . . The genius which was to penetrate the science of the age with a far more subtile science, to pass the bounds of space and time, venture into the dim spirit-realm, to attempt to establish a new religion in the world, began its letters in quarries and forges, in the smelting-pot and crucible, in ship-yards and dissecting-rooms. No one man is, perhaps, able to judge of the merits of his works on so many subjects. . . . It seems that he anticipated much science of the nineteenth century. . . . His superb speculation, as from a tower, over nature and arts, without ever losing sight of the texture and sequence of things, almost realizes his own picture in the *Principia* of the original integrity of man. . . . One of the missouriums and mastodons of literature, he is not to be measured by whole colleges of ordinary scholars. His stalwart presence would flutter the gowns of a university. Our books are false by being fragmentary. . . . But Swedenborg is systematic, and respective of the world in every sentence; all the means are orderly given; his faculties work with astronomic punctuality, and his admirable writing is pure from all pertness and egotism. He named his favorite views, the Doctrine of Forms, the Doctrine of Series and Degrees, the Doctrine of Influx, the Doctrine of Correspondence. His statement of these doctrines deserves to be studied in his books. Not every man can read them, but they will reward him who can. . . . His writings would be a sufficient library to a lonely and athletic student; and the *Economy of the Animal Kingdom* is one of those books which, by the sustained dignity of thinking, is an honor to the human race. . . . The *Animal Kingdom* is a book of wonderful merits. It was written with the highest end—to put science and the soul, long estranged from each other, at one again. . . . His religion thinks for him and is of universal application. He turns it on every side; it fits every part of life, interprets and dignifies every circumstance, . . . a teaching which accompanied him all day, . . . into his thinking, . . . into society, . . . into natural objects, . . . and opened the future world by indicating the continuity of the same laws. . . . That slow but commanding influence which he has acquired . . . must be excessive, . . . and have its tides before it subsides into a permanent amount."

Rev. Edwin Paxton Hood's estimate of Swedenborg:

"Swedenborg was one of the profoundest mathematicians of his age, a deep and acute thinker, a subtle logician, a various and versatile scholar—above all, a calm and most quiet bookman and penman, indisposed for any company, and never seen to court the company of the ignorant and the vulgar—ever the resort of the fanatic; a man of few words, until compelled to talk, or talking for a purpose; cool in temperament; never rocked by passion or impulse; always, as far as humanity can be, in equilibrium, weighing all his thoughts and all his actions; perpetually bent upon giving reasons for things; a man of strong inductive habits and powers, and consistent; a whole life of invariable rectitude. He was a Titan, and must take his place among the very highest and widest minds of our world."

Thomas Carlyle's estimate of Swedenborg:

"A man of great and indisputable cultivation, strong, mathematical intellect, and the most pious, seraphic turn of mind; a man beautiful, lovable, and tragical to me, with many thoughts in him which, when I interpret them for myself, I find to belong to the high and perennial in human thought. Whatever I may conjecture in my own defence about the strange impediments and unconquerable imprisoning conditions under which he had to live and to meditate, surely I am very far, indeed, from ranking him, or those that honestly follow him, under any dishonorable category."

Samuel Taylor Coleridge's estimate of Swedenborg:

"I can venture to assert that as a moralist Swedenborg is above all praise; and that as a naturalist, psychologist, and theologian he has strong and varied claims on the gratitude and admiration of the professional and philosophical student."

Henry James's estimate of Swedenborg:

"I fully concede to Swedenborg an extreme sobriety of mind displayed under all the exceptional circumstances of his career, and which ends by making us feel at last his every word to be almost insipid with veracity. I cordially appreciate, moreover, the rare destitution of wilfulness which characterizes all his researches; or, rather, the childlike docility of spirit which leads him to seek and to recognize, under all the most contradictory aspects of nature, the footsteps of the Highest.

"His books are a dry, unimpassioned, unexaggerated exposition of the things he daily saw and heard in the world of spirits, and of the spiritual laws which these things illustrate; with scarcely any effort whatever to blink the obvious outrage his experiences offer to sensuous prejudice, or to conciliate any interest in his reader which is not prompted by the latter's own original and unaffected relish of the truth. Such sincere books, it seems to me, were never before written."

An estimate of Swedenborg by the late Hon. Theophilus Parsons, for twenty-two years professor in the Cambridge Law School:

"I regard him as a man of remarkable ability and great and varied culture, taught, as no other man ever was taught, truths which no other man ever learned; and thus instructed that he might introduce among men a new system of truth or doctrine, excelling in character and exceeding in value any system of truth before known; a new gift, demanding, as the instrument by which it could be communicated, a man not only possessing extraordinary capacity and cultivation, but in both capacity and cultivation definitely adapted to the peculiar work he had to do."

APPENDIX B

Luther, Melancthon, and Calvin.*

"I have frequently conversed with these three leading Reformers of the Christian Church, and in that way have learned what the state of their life has been, from their first entrance into the spiritual world up to the present time."

LUTHER.

"As for Luther, from the time when he first went to the spiritual world he was a most vehement propagator and defender of his dogmas, and his zeal for them increased as the number of those from the earth who agreed with and favored him increased. A house was given him there like the one he had in the life of the body at Eisleben. In the centre of this house he erected a sort of throne, somewhat elevated, where he sat; he admitted hearers through the open door, and arranged them in order; nearest to himself he invited those who were the more favorable to him; behind them he placed those less favorable, and then he made speeches to them, occasionally permitting questions in order that he might obtain a kind of clew whereby to recommence the web of his discourse. Owing to this general favor, he at length imbibed a power of *persuasion*, which is so efficacious in the spiritual world that no one can

* Swedenborg's *True Christian Religion*, nos. 796–799.

resist it or speak against what is said. But as this was a kind of incantation used by the ancients, he was forbidden to speak from that power of persuasion any more; and after this, as before, he taught from the memory and understanding together. This power of persuasion, which is a kind of incantation, springs from self-love, owing to which it finally becomes of such a nature that when any one contradicts he not only attacks the subject in question, but also the person himself. This was the state of Luther's life up to the time of the last judgment, which took place in the spiritual world in the year 1757; but a year after that he was removed from his first house to another, and at the same time underwent a change of state. And in this state, having heard that I, who was in the natural world, spoke with those in the spiritual world, he, among others, came to me; and after some questions and answers he perceived that there is at this day an end of the former church and the beginning of a new church, of which Daniel prophesied, and which the Lord himself foretold in the evangelists; he also perceived that this new church was meant by the New Jerusalem in Revelation, and by the everlasting gospel which the angel flying in the midst of heaven preached to the inhabitants of the earth (xiv. 6). At this he became very angry and railed. But as he perceived that the new heaven (which was formed, and is still forming, of those who acknowledge the Lord alone as the God of heaven and earth, according to his words in Matt. xxviii. 18) [increased], and as he observed the number of his own congregations daily diminishing, he ceased his railing and came nearer to me, and began to talk with me more familiarly. And after he had been convinced that he had not derived his principal dogma of justification by faith alone from the Word, but from his own intelligence, he suffered himself to be instructed respecting the Lord, charity, true faith, free-will, and redemption also, and this exclusively from the Word. At length, after being convinced, he began to favor more and more those truths of which the new church is formed, and finally to confirm himself in them. At this time he was with me daily; and then, as often as he called those truths to mind, he began to laugh at his former dogmas as things diametrically opposed to the Word. I heard him say: 'Do not be surprised at my seizing upon justification by faith alone, excluding charity from its spiritual essence, also taking away from men all free-will in things spiritual, and affirming other things that depend on faith alone once accepted, as links on a chain, inasmuch as my object was to break away from the Roman Catholics, and this object I could not otherwise compass and attain. I, therefore, do not wonder at my own errors, but I do wonder that one crazy man could make so many others crazy.' As he said this he looked at some dogmatic writers beside him, men of celebrity in his time, faithful followers of his doctrine, who saw nothing contradictory to those dogmas in the sacred Scripture, although it does contradict them plainly. It was told me by the examining angels that this leader was in a state of conversion before many others who had confirmed themselves in the doctrine of justification by faith alone, because in his childhood, before he undertook the Reformation, he had imbibed the dogma of the pre-eminence of charity; and for this reason also, both in his writings and in his discourses, he taught charity so notably; and as a consequence, justifying faith with him was implanted in his external-natural man, but had not taken root in his internal-spiritual man.

It is otherwise, however, with those who in their childhood have confirmed themselves against the spirituality of charity, which also takes place of itself while justification by faith alone is being established by confirmations. I have conversed with the Prince of Saxony, with whom Luther had been associated in the world, and he told me that he had often upbraided Luther, especially for separating charity from faith, and declaring the latter to be saving and the former not, when, nevertheless, not only does the sacred Scripture unite those two universal means of salvation, but Paul also places charity before faith, when he says, 'And now abideth faith, hope, charity, these three; but the greatest of these is charity' (1 Cor. xiii. 13). But he said that Luther as often replied that he could not do otherwise, because of the Roman Catholics. This prince is among the happy."

MELANCTHON.

"As to what the lot of Melancthon was when he first entered the spiritual world, and what it was afterwards, I have been permitted to learn many things, not only from the angels, but also from himself, for I have conversed with him repeatedly—yet not so frequently as with Luther, nor so near to him. I have not conversed with him so frequently nor so near, because he could not approach me as Luther did, for the reason that he had given his exclusive attention to justification by faith alone, but not to charity; and I was surrounded by angelic spirits who were principled in charity, and they interfered with his approach to me. I heard that when he first entered the spiritual world a house was prepared for him like that in which he had dwelt in the world. This also takes place with the most of newcomers, owing to which they do not know but they are still in the natural world, and *the time elapsed since their death seems to them merely as a sleep.* Everything in his room was also like what he formerly had: he had the same kind of a table, the same kind of a secretary with drawers, and also the same kind of a library; so that as soon as he came there, as if he had just awakened from a sleep, he seated himself at the table and continued his writing, and that, too, on the subject of justification by faith alone, and so on for several days, saying nothing whatever about charity. The angels, perceiving this, asked him through messengers why he did not write about charity also. He replied that there was nothing belonging to the church in charity, for if it were to be received as in any way an essential principle of the church, man would also attribute to himself the merit of justification, and consequently of salvation, and thus he would also rob faith of its spiritual essence. When the angels who were over his head perceived this, and when the angels who were associated with him when he was outside of his house heard it, they all withdrew; for angels are associated with every new-comer at the beginning. A few weeks after this occurrence the things that he used in his room began to be obscured and at length to disappear, until at last there was nothing left there but the table, paper, and inkstand; and, moreover, the walls of his room seemed to be plastered with lime, and the floor to be covered with yellow bricks, and his clothing to become coarser. Wondering at this, he inquired of those about him why it was so; and he was told that it was because he had removed charity from the church, which was, nevertheless, its heart. But as he often denied this, and again commenced to write about faith as the one only essential of the church, and the means of salvation, and to remove charity more and more, he suddenly seemed to himself to be under ground in a certain prison, where there were others like him. And when he wished to go out he was detained, and it was announced to him that no other lot awaited those who thrust charity and good works outside of the doors of the church. But inasmuch as he had been one of the Reformers of the church, he was released from that prison by the Lord's command, and sent back to his former room, where there was nothing but the table, paper, and ink-stand. But still, owing to his confirmed ideas, he bedaubed the paper with the same error, so that he could not be kept from being alternately sent down to his captive fellows and sent back again. When sent back, he appeared in a garment made of a hairy skin, because faith without charity is cold. He told me himself that there was another room adjoining his own in the rear, in which there were three tables, at which sat men like himself, who had also exiled charity, and that a fourth table also sometimes appeared there, on which were seen monstrous things in various forms, by which, however, they were not frightened from their work. He said that he conversed with these others, and was confirmed by them daily. After some time, however, incited by fear, he began to write something about charity; but what he wrote on the paper one day he did not see the next; for this happens to every one there when he commits anything to paper from the external man only, and not at the same time from the internal, thus from compulsion and not from freedom. It is obliterated of itself. But after the establishment by the Lord of the new heaven was begun, by the light from this heaven he began to think that perhaps he might be in error; so that, owing to anxiety about his lot, he felt impressed upon him some interior ideas respecting charity. In this state he consulted the Word, and then his eyes were opened, and he saw that it was all filled with *love to God and love to the neighbor,* so that it was as the Lord says: on these two commandments hang the law and the prophets, that is, the whole Word. From this time he was transferred more interiorly to the southwest, and so to another house, from which he conversed with me, saying that his writings on charity did not then disappear as formerly, but appeared obscurely the next day. One thing I wondered at, that when he walked his steps had a striking sound, like those of a man walking with iron heels on a stone pavement. To this must be added that when any novitiate from the world entered his room to talk with him or see him, he would summon one from among spirits given to magic, who by fantasy could call up various beautiful shapes, and who then adorned his chamber with ornaments and flowered tapestry, and also with the appearance of a library in the centre. As soon as the visitors were gone, however, these shapes vanished, and the former plastering and emptiness returned. But this was when he was in his former state."

CALVIN

"Of Calvin I have heard the following: 1. When he first went to the spiritual world he would not believe but that he was still in the world where he was born; and although he heard from the angels associated with him first in order that he was then in their world, and not in his former one, he said, 'I have the same body, the same hands, and similar senses.' But the angels instructed him to the effect that he was then in a substantial body, and that he was formerly not only in that same body, but also in a material one, which invested the substantial; and that the material body had been cast off, the substantial body, from which a man is a man, remaining. This he at first understood; but the day afterwards he returned to his former belief, that he was still in the world where he was born. This was because he was a sensual man, having no belief but what he could draw from the objects of the bodily senses; from this arose the fact that all the dogmas of his faith were conclusions drawn from his self-derived intelligence, and not from the Word. His quoting the Word was in order to win the assent of the common people. 2. After this first period, the angels having left him, he wandered about inquiring for those who in ancient times believed in predestination; and he was told that they had been removed from that place, and shut up and covered over, and there was no way open to them except in a backward direction under the earth; but that the disciples of Godeschalk still went about freely, and sometimes assembled in a place called, in spiritual language, *Pyris*. And as he longed for their company, he was conducted to an assembly where some of them were standing; and when he came among them he was in his heart's delight, and bound himself to them by interior friendship. 3. But after the followers of Godeschalk were led away to their brethren in the cavern Calvin became tired; he, therefore, sought here and there for an asylum, and was finally received into a certain society, composed wholly of simple-minded persons, some of whom were also religious; and when he saw that they knew nothing about predestination, and could not understand anything about it, he betook himself to one corner of the society, and there hid himself for a long time; nor did he open his mouth on any ecclesiastical subject. This was providential, in order that he might withdraw from his error respecting predestination, and that the ranks of those who after the Synod of Dort adhered to that detestable heresy might be filled up; they were all gradually sent away to their fellows in the cavern. 4. At length it was asked by the modern Predestinarians, Where is Calvin? And after a search he was found on the confines of a certain society consisting exclusively of simple-minded persons. He was, therefore, called away from there, and conducted to a certain governor who was filled with similar dregs. This governor, therefore, took him into his house and guarded him, and this until the new heaven began to be established by the Lord; and then, as his guardian governor was cast out together with his troop, Calvin betook himself to a certain house of harlotry, and remained there for some time. 5. And as he then enjoyed the liberty of wandering about, and also of coming near to the place where I was stopping, I was permitted to converse with him. At first I spoke of the new heaven which at this day is being formed by those who acknowledge the Lord alone as the God of heaven and earth, according to his words in Matt. xxviii. 18. I told him that they believe that He and the Father are one (John x. 30), that He is in the Father and the Father in Him, that whosoever sees and knows Him sees and knows the Father also (John xiv. 6–11), and that thus there is one God in the church as in heaven. At first, when I said this, he was as usual silent; but after half an hour he broke the silence and said: 'Was not Christ a man, the son of Mary, the wife of Joseph? How can a man be worshipped as God?' I answered, 'Is not Jesus Christ, our Redeemer and Saviour, both God and man?' He replied, 'He is both God and man; nevertheless the divinity is not his, but the Father's.' I asked, 'Where, then, is Christ?' He answered, 'In the lowest parts of heaven, as He proved by his humiliation before the Father and by suffering himself to be crucified.' To this he added some witty remarks about the worship of Him, which then broke forth from the world into his memory, the sum of which was, that the worship of Christ was nothing but idolatry, and he wanted to add something horrible about that worship; but the angels who were with me shut his lips. But I, being zealous to convert him, said, 'The Lord our Saviour is not only both God and Man, but in Him, moreover, God is Man and Man is God.' And this I confirmed by Paul's saying, 'That in Him dwelleth all the fulness of divinity bodily' (Col. ii. 9); and by John's, 'That He is the true God and eternal life' (1 Epistle v. 20); as also from the words of the Lord himself, 'That it is the will of the Father that whosoever believes on the Son hath eternal life, and that he who believes not shall not see life, but the wrath of God abideth on him' (John iii. 36; vi. 40); and, finally, by what is called the Athanasian Creed, which declares that in Christ, God and Man are not two but one, and are in one Person, like the soul and body in man. Hearing this, he replied: 'What are all those things which you have presented from the Word but empty sounds? Is not the Word the book of all heresies, and so like the weathercocks on housetops and ships' masts, which turn every way according to the wind? It is *predestination alone* that determines all things pertaining to religion; this is the habitation and tabernacle where they all meet; and faith, through which come justification and salvation, is there the innermost place and sanctuary. Has any man free-will in spiritual things? Is not the whole of salvation gratuitous? Any arguments, therefore, against these principles, and so against predestination, I listen to and value as much as I do eructations from the stomach or the rumbling of the bowels. Hence I have thought that a temple wherein they teach anything else from the Word, and the crowd there congregated, are like a pen of beasts containing both sheep and wolves, the latter being muzzled, however, by the laws of civil justice, lest they should attack the sheep (by the sheep I mean the predestined); and I regard the preaching and praying there like so much hiccoughing. But I will give you my confession of faith; it is this: There is a God, and He is omnipotent; and there is no salvation for any but those who are elected and predestined to heaven by God the Father; and all others are condemned to their lot, that is, to their fate.' Hearing this, I retorted, with much warmth, 'What you say is impious. Begone, wicked spirit! Since you are in the spiritual world, do you not know there is a heaven and a hell, and that predestination involves that some are enrolled for heaven and some for hell? Can you, then, form to yourself any other idea of God than as of a tyrant, who admits His favorites into the city and sends the rest to the rack? You ought to be ashamed of yourself.' I then read to him what is written in the dogmatic book of the evangelical Protestants, called Formula Concordiæ, about the erroneous doctrine of the Calvinists respecting the worship of the Lord and predestination. Respecting the worship of the Lord, as follows: 'It is damnable idolatry, if the confidence and faith of the heart are placed in Christ, not only according to his divine, but also according to his human, nature, and the honor of worship is directed to both.' And respecting predestination, as follows: 'Christ did not die for all men, but only for the elect. God has created the greater part of men for eternal damnation, and does not wish that this part should be converted and live. The elect and born again cannot lose faith and the Holy Spirit, although they should commit all kinds of great sins and crimes. But those who are not elected are necessarily damned, nor can they attain to salvation even if they were to be baptized a thousand times, to partake of the sacrament daily, and, moreover, to lead as holy and blameless a life as it is ever possible to live' (from the Leipsic edition of 1756, pp. 837, 838). After reading this, I asked him whether this which was written in that book was from his doctrine or not. He said that it was, but that he did not remember whether or not those very words had flowed from his pen, although they might have flowed from his lips. All the servants of the Lord hearing this, withdrew from him, and he betook himself hastily to a way that led to a cave which is occupied by those who have confirmed in themselves the execrable dogma of predestination. I afterwards conversed with some of those imprisoned in that cave and asked about their lot. They said that they were compelled to labor for food, that all were enemies of each other, that each sought an occasion to do evil to the other, and also did it whenever he found the slightest opportunity, and that this was the delight of their lives. On predestination and the predestinarians, see also what is said above, n. 485-488.

"I have also conversed with many others, both with followers of these three men and with heretics [or other sects]; and respecting all of them I was enabled to form this conclusion: that whoever among them have lived a life of charity, and still more those who have loved truth because it is truth, in the spiritual world suffer themselves to be instructed, and accept the doctrines of the new church; while, on the other hand, those who have confirmed themselves in falsities of religion, and also those who have lived an evil life, do not suffer themselves to be instructed. These latter remove step by step from the new heaven, and associate themselves with their like who are in hell, where they confirm themselves more and more obstinately against the worship of the Lord, even to such an extent that they cannot bear to hear the name of Jesus. But it is the reverse in heaven, where all unanimously acknowledge the Lord as the God of heaven."

THE END

By JULIAN RALPH

By JULIAN RALPH—*Continued*

OUR GREAT WEST. A Study of the Present Conditions and Future Possibilities of the New Commonwealths and Capitals of the United States. Illustrated. 8vo, Cloth, $2 50.

The vivid descriptions, careful statistics, and thoroughly earnest and conscientious spirit of this book make it well worthy the attention of all American students of economics. —*Zion's Herald*, Boston.

"Our Great West" is marked by a splendid vigor of description.—*The Sun*, N. Y.

It supplies a need, for no one else has covered the ground so thoroughly or so satisfactorily.—*Critic*, N. Y.

ON CANADA'S FRONTIER. Sketches of History, Sport, and Adventure; and of the Indians, Missionaries, Fur-traders, and Newer Settlers of Western Canada. Illustrated. 8vo, Cloth, $2 50.

The articles are not statistical, they are rather a series of bright and often humorous sketches of the odd characters and scenes that accompany the settlement of a new country, with accounts of the adventures which the author and the artist, Mr. Remington, had on their hunting and fishing tours.—*Book Buyer*, N. Y.

HARPER & BROTHERS, PUBLISHERS

NEW YORK AND LONDON

☞ *Any of the above works will be sent by mail, postage prepaid, to any part of the United States, Canada, or Mexico, on receipt of the price.*

Published by

Facsimile Publisher
Ashok Vihar, Delhi-110052 (India)
Website: www.facsimilepublisher.com

Distributed by

Gyan Books Pvt. Ltd.
5, Ansari Road, Daryaganj, New Delhi-110002 (India)
E-mail: books@gyanbooks.com, Website: www.gyanbooks.com

2 222000 013233